BROKEN CONNECTIONS

The little boy and the old man

Said the little boy, "Sometimes I drop my spoon."
Said the little old man, "I do that too."
The little boy whispered, "I wet my pants."
"I do that too," laughed the little old man.
Said the little boy, "I often cry."
The old man nodded, "So do I."
"But worst of all," said the boy, "it seems
Grown-ups don't pay attention to me."
And he felt the warmth of a wrinkled old hand.
"I know what you mean," said the little old man.

Shel Silverstein

From: *A light in the Attic,*
poems and drawings by Shel Silverstein,
HarperCollins Publishers, 1981

LIDUIN SOUREN & EMILE FRANSSEN

Broken
Connections

ALZHEIMER'S DISEASE

PART II – PRACTICAL GUIDELINES FOR CARING
FOR THE ALZHEIMER PATIENT

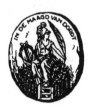

SWETS & ZEITLINGER B.V.   PUBLISHERS

LISSE ∎ BERWYN, PA

Library of Congress Cataloging-in-Publication Data

Souren, Liduïn
    [Verbroken verbindingen. English]
    Broken connections : Alzheimer's disease / Liduïn Souren & Emile Franssen.
      p.   cm.
    Includes bibliographical references.
    Contents: pt. 1. Origin and course -- pt2. Practical guidelines for caring for the
Alzheimer patient.
    ISBN 90 265 1334 8 (pt 1). -- ISBN 90 265 13712 (pt. 2)
    1. Alzheimer's disease. 2. Alzheimer's disease--Patients--Care. I. Franssen, Emile
II. Title.
    [DNLM: 1. Alzheimer's disease. WM 220s724v 1993a]
    RC523.S6813 1993
    616.8'31--dc20
    DNLM/DLC   93-25579
    for Library of Congress   CIP

CIP-gegevens Koninklijke Bibliotheek, Den Haag

Souren, Liduïn
Broken connections : Alzheimer's disease / Liduïn Souren & Emile Franssen; [transl. from the
Dutch: R.M.J. van der Wilden-Fall]. – Lisse [etc.] : Swets & Zeitlinger
Pt.II: Practical guidelines for caring for the Alzheimer patient.
Vert van: Verbroken verbindingen : de ziekte van Alzheimer. Dl.II: Praktische richtlijnen voor
het omgaan met de Alzheimer-patient. Amsterdam [etc.], 1993
Met lit. opg., reg.
ISBN 90-265-1371-2
NUGI 759
Trefw.: ziekte van Alzheimer

Translation: R.M.J. van der Wilden-Fall, MBE, MA (Oxon)
Cover design: Rob Molthoff, LineaForma, Alkmaar
Cover printed in the Netherlands by Casparie, IJsselstein
Printed in the Netherlands by Offsetdrukkerij Kanters B.V., Alblasserdam

ISBN 90 265 1371 2
NUGI 759

TO OUR PARENTS

FOREWORD

Twenty years ago, Alzheimer's disease was known to only a handful of professionals. It is now a familiar term in most households in the United States. No disease is more dreaded. The loss of cognitive function associated with Alzheimer's disease represents the worst fear of old age. Alzheimer's disease conjures up the image of a loved elderly relative, alive but unable to participate in even the rudimentary activities associated with family life. The disease poses the burden of long and arduous caregiving and constitutes the most profound personal and family tragedy. It taxes the skills of the most experienced and dedicated professional and raises the most basic questions about the benefits and burdens of care.

Over five million Americans are afflicted withe Alzheimer's disease. Yet an astounding number of health care professionals and family caregivers lack even rudimentary information about the disease: its underlying cause, the progression of symptoms, and perhaps most importantly, strategies for interacting with patients and their families. Very few comprehensive sources of information about Alzheimer's disease are available to family members and health care professionals. This text by Liduïn Souren and Emile Franssen is a major step in rectifying this deficiency.

The impetus for the book came from the autors' familiarity with the care provided in residential home settings and in nursing homes in the United States and in Holland. Liduïn Souren has extensive experience as a teacher and consultant in geriatric nursing. Emile Franssen, a neurologist, is internationally recognized for his research and clinical expertise in dementia and Alzheimer's disease. In their capacity as researchers, consultants and educators, they have observed that professional and non professional care givers working with patients with cognitive disorders lack basic information about strategies for managing the behavioral manifestations of Alzheimer's disease. They have found staff highly responsive to their suggestions for managing patients. And, most importantly, they have seen first hand the improvements which can be achieved when patients' dysfunctions are adequately assessed, understood and remediated.

The book, which is also published in the Netherlands, is divided into two parts. Part I explores the notion of dementia and its causes. As can only be done when one has extensive knowledge, the authors are able to distill the essence of the disease and present it's pathophysiology in a form which is at the same time comprehensive and easy to understand. Appropriately titled *Broken Connections*, Part I juxtaposes the behavioral manifestations of Alzheimer's disease with the underlying neurologic pathology. So, for example, absent-mindedness, disturbances of day-night rhythm and "sundowning" are explained within the context of the concomitant neurologic deficits.

Part II of *Broken Connections* focuses on practical guidelines and is meant for the primary caregiver of Alzheimer's patients. The content delineates four stages which represent the progressive loss of function associated with the disease. For each stage, the authors provide a scheme of practical suggestions for managing socio-recreational function, household and daily personal care and hygiene. Included in this *LIMIT scheme* is a *LIMIT test* which poses questions which objectively determine what patients are able to do. The LIMIT scheme offers practical suggestions for preserving existing function. In Stage I of the disease, for example a discussion about handling money provides questions to determine the degree to which patients can handle money: can the patient distinguish between less, much and more? Can he name coins and bills and distinguish the different values? Specific suggestions for helping patients manage money include encouraging the patient to pay at the check-out and sort change at home or stack similar coins.

The book is perfused with the authors' enthusiasm for improving care for patients with Alzheimer's disease. Their intent is to tell the reader that the patients' behavior can be understood and that there exists a wide repertoire of activities which can preserve the patient's function and slow the slope of decline. By sharing their own and other's expertise, this book diminishes the isolation of countless millions of caregivers faced with the daily task of improving the lives of Alzheimer's patients.

Mathy Mezey, Ed.D., F.A.A.N.
Independence Foundation Professor of Nursing Educaton
New York University

PREFACE

The authors of this book are both very concerned with the lot of Alzheimer patients and their immediate caregivers. Through her work as a tutor of nursing and geriatrics Liduin Souren has repeatedly come across many unanswered questions from those most closely involved in caring for the patients. Her husband, Emile Franssen, is engaged on scientific research into the neurological aspects of Alzheimer's disease. From the background of his know-how as a neurologist/psychiatrist he explains the working of the brain and the connection between the brain and behavior in a readily understandable way. Many of the questions concerning the uncomprehended behavior of the Alzheimer patient come up for discussion and become clear to the attentive reader. Attention is also paid to psychological factors which influence behavior.

Part II deals comprehensively with the "treatment". On the basis of the theoretical model from Part I indications are given on the way in which the patient's daily life can be structured. Clear and conveniently arranged schemes show how the caregiver can approach the patient in a manner which makes use of the possibilities still available, whereby life becomes more bearable both for the patient and also for the caregiver.

Amongst the many books on these subjects which have appeared during the last few years, these two books certainly deserve a place for their clarity, comprehensiveness and the lucidity of the schemes.

The DUTCH ALZHEIMER FOUNDATION is very pleased that these two compatriots, who live and work in New York, have made their experience and knowledge accessible to us.

H.W. ter Haar, M.D., Secretary Dutch Alzheimer Foundation
A.S.H. van Moll, Former Director Dutch Alzheimer Foundation

CONTENTS

INTRODUCTION

Part I of our book *Broken Connections. Alzheimer's Disease* contains a description of various aspects of Alzheimer's disease (Part I: Origin and Course). This description shows how in the course of this illness a preliminary stage and four successive stages of ever increasing loss of previously learned activities and mastered skills can be distinguished. One of the characteristics of this disease is the gradual disorganization and finally the total loss of initiative and purposive movement. This leads to increasing personal neglect. The caregiver wants to keep the patient active as long as possible by involving him as much as he can in all activities. But how much is 'as much as possible'? What determines whether and to what extent the patient in a specific phase can still actively participate in an activity? That is mainly determined by the complexity of that activity. All activities which require insight, overview, preparation and assessment soon become impossible. Later on the simpler actions also become too difficult.

In Part II we give a systematic survey of the functions, i.e. all ever learned activities, which are lost in the course of the illness. The emphasis is on what the patient can indeed still do. The course of the illness has been divided into four stages, which are marked by the loss of a specific function. Practical guidelines and suggestions are given as to how to keep a patient as busy as possible and how to be constructively occupied with him or her. After the schemes a questionnaire (the LIMIT test) has been included, by means of which the caregiver can determine to what extent the patient can still manage on his own. This makes it easier for the caregiver to establish the phase of the illness in which the patient finds himself and to provide more tailor-made help.

Stages
In the preliminary stage of Alzheimer's disease the patient already has great problems in carrying out his professional activities. In stage I (stimulation

stage) the performance of household activities, which call for planning and insight, also becomes impossible. Insight into financial affairs is lacking and the patient has to be placed under tutelage. He can no longer spend his time meaningfully without help and can no longer mix with other people on an equal footing. In this stage the patient has to be encouraged to carry out the daily routine activities of personal hygiene at the appropriate time.

In stage II of the illness (intervention stage) the state of helplessness in the contact with other people is already such that most patients are now unable to hold their own. The inability to express themselves adequately often plays a part here. The caregiver determines the choice of activities and takes the initiative. Recreational activities should preferably be directed to stimulating functions which have not yet been entirely lost. Most household activities have become too complex, but the patient can still perform the separate component actions himself, under the supervision and with the encouragement of the caregiver and often to his own enjoyment. The daily personal hygiene also requires supervision and supervisory care is now necessary 24 hours a day.

Stage III (partial take-over of activities by the caregiver) is principally characterized by the gradual loss of realization of the concept of ones own body, of the relationship between the parts of the body and of the relationship of the body to the environment. Partly as a result of this it becomes impossible to independently perform the routine activities of personal hygiene and the patient is only able to perform component actions, with the constant supervision and sometimes the actual help of the caregiver. Every movement becomes disorganized, lacks purpose and rapidly comes to a standstill or is continually repeated. About halfway through this stage the patient loses his ability to cope with going to the toilet. Later on he is no longer able to react appropriately upon the urge to urinate or defecate. For his environment this is often totally unacceptable. Incontinence is often the most compelling reason for nursing home placement. The patient now requires continual care. Stage III has therefore been divided into two phases: in phase III-A the patient still has control of his toilet activities, but in phase III-B he is incontinent.

In stage IV of the illness (total take-over of activities) the last vestiges of the power of verbal expression are lost. This stage is also characterized by the gradual loss of all movement and the initiative to move. This stage is divided into five phases: A, B, C, D and E. In phase A the patient loses all power of speech, but he can still walk on his own. In phase B he can no longer walk, but can still stand (with support) and sit up. In phase C he cannot sit up any longer, but can still move his head. In phase D the latter movement has also become impossible, but he can sometimes move his arms. In phase E he cannot do this any longer. He occasionally opens his eyes as a reaction to bright light or to being loudly addressed. He still reacts to pain, either with groans or shrieks. He can only swallow very slowly, but the swallowing reflex, just as the coughing reflex, often remains intact for a long time.

The final phase is characterized by total immobility: all urge to move has ceased and even strong external stimuli no longer alter the situation. Many patients do not reach the last phase of the illness and die from an additional disorder.

LIMIT Scheme and LIMIT Test

Thus the possibilities for the caregiver of doing things together with the patient gradually become more restricted. In the first two stages of the illness these possibilities are still considerable and even in the later stages they are not entirely exhausted. The *LIMIT scheme* is intended as a practical guide for the caregiver in the daily contact with the Alzheimer patient in each of the stages mentioned above. The activities are subdivided into three groups: socio-recreational, household and daily personal care and hygiene activities.

First an indication is given of the activities or actions with which the patient only needs encouragement. This is followed by a description of the activities or actions where the caregiver has actively to intervene. Then come the activities or actions where the caregiver has partially or totally to take over from the patient. Finally an indication is given of the best attitude for the caregiver to adopt in order to achieve the desired result. This is particularly important in dealing with factors such as anxiety, resistence or agression in the patient, which are obstacles to a smooth execution of the intended activities. By letting the patient do the LIMIT test, the caregiver can form an idea of the nature of the problems which the patient has with the various activities.

The basic consideration for the caregiver is always: *how can the patient be kept active as long as possible?* What can the patient still do, with or without help, and if he needs help, how much and what with? Each individual patient has other possibilities and needs. One patient can do certain things which another patient definitely can not. This applies in particular to the socio-recreational activities. The LIMIT scheme therefore gives a number of concrete alternatives, from which the caregiver can make a choice.

From what has been said above, it follows that it is not possible to establish from isolated preserved activities which stage of the illness the patient is now in. There can be various reasons why a patient can no longer perform a particular action or activity. It can happen, for instance, that a patient in stage I can no longer wash himself because of arthritis in the joints. Another patient may already be incontinent in stage II as a result of stress incontinence or cystitis.

In caring for dementing people the nature of the interaction between patient and caregiver, the extent to which the caregiver succeeds in establishing contact with the patient, is of the greatest importance for a successful engagement of the patient.

The authors hope that this book can make a contribution to achieving this contact, so as to make the life of the Alzheimer patient and his caregiver more bearable.

CHAPTER I

THE FIRST SYMPTOMS

More than half of all the patients with dementia suffer from Alzheimer's disease. Nevertheless there can be great difficulties involved in making the diagnosis. Frequently someone with behavioral and memory disturbances first pays a visit, accompanied by a worried spouse, son, daughter or close friend, to his own doctor. Having assessed the situation, the doctor will refer him to the specialist. Nowadays the diagnosis is often made by a team of specialists, consisting of a psychiatrist, a neurologist, a geriatrician, a psychologist, a social worker and a nurse. This multidisciplinary approach offers the greatest guarantee of not being too late in establishing treatable causes of memory disturbances, such as depression or certain somatic disorders.

Unfortunately there is still no specific test for diagnosing Alzheimer's disease. Particularly the stage of incipient illness it is usually very difficult to make the diagnosis with any degree of certainty. As a rule the patient has to pay regular visits and undergo repeated tests, before the characteristic pattern of disturbed memory, disturbed cognitive powers, loss of function and subtle personality changes becomes evident. This pattern, which was outlined in the last chapters of Part I, comes up for further discussion in the following chapters and is taken as the starting point for determining the activities which the patient can still perform, either independently or with adjusted assistance.

It must be stressed, that this pattern gives a broad description of the course of Alzheimer's disease. Not every patient always exhibits exactly the same picture; there are individual differences. Thus, for example, there are patients who can no longer walk on their own, but can still speak; there are patients who can still walk, but can no longer eat with a spoon.

If the loss of function in the patient, who has been diagnosed as suffering from Alzheimer, does not happen in accordance with the pattern, however, there could be other, treatable causes. Thus it is possible that the Alzheimer patient, who can no longer walk on his own, but can still speak in sentences, may have arthritis of the hips, be subject to side effects of medication, have swollen ankles or loss of feeling in the feet resulting from disorders of the peripheral nerves of the legs. The patient himself is unable to make this clear.

But in broad outline the course of the loss of function is predictable and happens according to the pattern: what was learnt last, is the first to be lost. It is always important to ensure that a particular loss of function is not automatically ascribed to the Alzheimer process. All sorts of complications can lead to a premature loss of function. The LIMIT scheme described in the following chapters, which is based on what the patient can do himself, is intended as a guideline for the caregiver.

The preliminary stage of Alzheimer's disease
The first symptoms of incipient Alzheimer's disease are vague, so that later on it is difficult to indicate when it all began. Whether and when these subtle behavioral changes in the person are noticed by those around him, partly depends on the way in which he is actively involved in the world and how complicated that world is. It is noticeable that he loses the ability to apply his acquired knowledge in situations which are unfamiliar. For instance, he cannot learn to cope with new materials and tools. He can no longer improvise and cannot find new solutions to old problems. He loses his creativity and security. That is why he avoids new and unknown situations, becomes extremely cautious and creates an impression of indecision and sometimes of refusal to work.

The loss of mental functions first becomes evident under stress. The more responsibilities a person has and the more complicated his work, the greater the chance of stress. Many healthy older people have more difficulty in coping with the continual tensions of their work than younger people. This applies all the more to people in the initial stages of dementia.

In the beginning of Alzheimer's disease the stress tolerance declines. Even in routine situations, which were not preceded by extra stress, efficiency in action is on the decrease: the patient can no longer cope with his work and makes an increasing number of mistakes. Work which he has done all his life without any problems, now becomes too difficult for him to complete. He can no longer concentrate effectively and is more quickly distracted. He forgets important appointments. He can no longer use his time efficiently and no longer organize and plan his scheme of work. If this situation goes on long enough, his colleagues become aware of it and he gets problems with his employer. Incapacity for work leads to early retirement.

There are also problems at home. Subtle changes of personality occur. The patient loses his interest in his hobbies, exhibits less initiative and interest in his environment and becomes more passive. He seems less interested in other people, takes less account of their feelings, even with those of his (marriage) partner and his friends. He loses his curiosity in what is happening in the world and no longer has any enthusiasm for anything. He is still aware in broad lines of important matters in which he is personally involved, such as in the family, but he cannot remember any details.

Events in which he is emotionally involved are easier for him to remember than objective facts which have no emotional appeal. If he reads a newspaper or magazine, at the end of the paragraph he no longer knows what he has read. His mental scope quickly shrinks. But he also begins to have problems with the organization of his more direct living space. He becomes untidier, continually forgets where he has put his personal belongings, which can lead to panic if it happens to be his purse or latchkey.

His experience of time as an orderly succession of moments also becomes disturbed and he more often forgets what day of the week it is and what time of day. This makes it difficult for him to estimate time properly. It can happen that one day, perhaps after a short period of heightened stress, he suddenly gets hopelessly lost in surroundings which are unknown to him and is panic stricken, because he no longer knows how he got there. That not infrequently happens for the first time when he is on holiday abroad; he is then suddenly confronted with an unknown environment, where the people speak an unknown language. The extra stress of the journey and the unknown environment are enough to make him disoriented.

The initially almost imperceptible loss of cognitive functions can sometimes suddenly and dramatically become manifest. It seems as though the illness has suddenly started, but careful questioning shows that this is not so. The following case history is an example of this.

A 56-year-old dentist visited the memory clinic. A few weeks before he had been standing in front of one of his patients who was seated in the dentist's chair. He picked up an instrument from the table and suddenly no longer knew why he had picked it up and what he was supposed to do with it. Somewhat shocked and embarrassed, he apologized to the patient and had to stop the session. He thought he must be overtired, as he had just had a few very busy days, in which he had worked on until late in the evening. When, after a few days' rest, he was again confronted with the same problem, he was really worried and went to see a doctor, thinking that he had perhaps had a slight stroke. However, a neurological examination did not reveal any abnormality. At the memory clinic an extensive and detailed examination of his mental functions showed unmistakable signs of a memory defect, of which neither he nor his wife were aware. On further questioning his wife reported that he had for some time been irritated by the fact that his dental technician repeatedly delivered dentures which turned out not to fit. It now became clear that the mistake had been made by the dentist himself, who had mixed up the patients' dental impressions. The dentist was unable to resume his work and had to give up his practice.

The patient in the preliminary stage of the disease is no longer able to take responsible decisions on important matters, because he is unable to conjure up all possible details of a situation, or because he devotes excessive attention to one single detail. He cannot weigh up the alternatives, cannot make a well-considered choice and cannot take an overall view of the consequences of a decision. This often leads to injudicious management of finances or irresponsibly giving money away. Generally speaking his actions become more impulsive and less critical and well-considered.

His behavior, in particular towards his spouse, shows signs of a lack of consideration and of inattention. He seems to concern himself less with things which affect them both. He is often querulous and has periods during which he sits brooding. He leans increasingly on his partner and accepts less and less responsibility himself. At the same time he may become argumentative with his partner. His behavior sometimes resembles that of a tiresome teenager. He asks a question and keeps on repeating it, because he forgets that he had already asked it and because he has forgotten the answer. Sometimes he gets cross with somebody who draws attention to this. He evidently views coming events such as engagements or visits with anxious anticipation. The patient keeps on asking his partner: "Shouldn't we be going now?" "When are we going?" He cannot cope with having to wait and it makes him agitated. He can not make even a simple decision independently. He has a vague and indefinable feeling of anxiety, of some-thing that is going to happen in an uncertain future, something he doesn't know about and over which he has no control. In particular this loss of control over the situation is very frustrating to him. Sometimes he tries to find explanations for his anxiety, such as a worrying financial or health situation, which according to him is sure to arise in the near future.

Indeterminable feelings of agitation and impatience also lead to an increased urge to move and to periodical restlessness in order to work off the tension.

All these problems bear witness to the beginning of disorientation, of inability to determine ones own course, and of increasing helplessness. Every patient tries in his or her own individual way to make sense of his changed world. Often he denies both to himself and to other people that anything is the matter. In this early stage of the illness the partner will also often deny everything and react irritably to the patient's difficult behavior, which he cannot understand. Increasing tension builds up between the patient and his partner, thus disturbing their relationship. For the patient as well as for the partner one of the great problems of this disease is the imbalance between a comparatively undisturbed level of energy and the possibilities of making this energy productive. If the of energy cannot be converted into constructive activities, then it can only have a destructive effect. This conduct is also reminiscent of the behavior of children and young teenagers. Being confronted with ones own incapacity leads moreover to waxing and waning feelings of depression and a loss of the feeling of self-respect.

In essence the care of the Alzheimer patient consists to a great extent in structurizing his world: the daily arrangement and simplification of his activities. Allowing the patient to do as far as possible what he enjoys doing, increases his sense of self-esteem. To confront an Alzheimer patient with his loss of memory and mental powers is like reminding a blind man of the loss of his eyes, or someone with an amputation of the loss of his limb. The less he is confronted with his defect, the less his sense of self-respect is affected by it. Encouragement and compliments help combat feelings of depression.

If recreational activities are attuned to the patient's mental grasp, he can put his energy to productive use. After all, from the point of view of society he is no longer productive and has no further responsibility towards society. He only has to see to it that he fills his time constructively, but even that is impossible without help. For him being busy in the recreational sense is always being busy with the other person, his partner, on a level of equality and in attunement with the interests and capacities he still possesses. Games are a good means of contact, a link with another person and with the world around him. A game forms a distraction from his feelings of fear and agitation. It is important that he is taken seriously in the game, regardless of whether he does something perfectly or not. Even daily activities can be performed as a game, provided the partners trust one another and one partner does not appear to be outsmarting the other and does not over-emphasize who lays down the rules.

The following four chapters, one for each subsequent stage of the disease, contain schemes in which an indication is given of the points to which the caregiver must pay extra attention in the relevant stage. The group of activities is mentioned at the top of each page, such as *Financial and Legal Affairs (General)*. For an overview see the following pages.

The scheme shows subsequently:
– what part of these activities the patient can actually still do himself;
– where he needs stimulation, but can further do it himself;
– in which activities the caregiver has to intervene;
– which activities have to be partially taken over by the caregiver;
– which activities have to be totally taken over by the caregiver.

At the beginning of each chapter a brief explanation is given of the accumulated functional loss of the patient, his experience of this loss and the way he may try to cope.

Stage I – The stimulation stage	Stage II – The intervention stage

Financial and legal affairs

General 34	
Getting a handle on money 36	Getting a handle on money 79

Social and recreational activities

Driving a car 38	Receiving guests 80
Receiving guests 39	In the garden 81
Telephoning 41	Hobbies and games 82
Pets 42	Broken words connection game 84
The garden 43	Games and puzzles 86
Hobbies 44	Music and singing 87
Broken words connection game 46	Making collages 88
	Drawing, coloring, painting 90
	Clay modeling 91
	Construction components 92
	Outside activities 93
	Swimming, aquatic gymnastics 94
	(Folk)dancing 96
	Ball games 98
	Rope games 99
	Hoop games 100
	Club games 101

Household

General 48	General 102
Shopping 51	Shopping 104
Kitchen activities 52	Kitchen activities 105

Personal care and hygiene

Body scheme 54	Body scheme 108
Bathing and skin care 56	Bathing and skin care 110
Hand care 58	Hand care 112
Foot care 59	Foot care 113
Oral and dental care 60	Oral and dental care 114
Facial care 62	Facial care 116
Clothing 64	Clothing 118
Eating and drinking 66	Eating and drinking 120
Going to the toilet 68	Going to the toilet 123

CHAPTER 2

STAGE I

SUPERVISION AND STIMULATION

In the first stage of the disease the mental functions become disturbed in such a way that the patient can no longer cope alone with his personal and domestic affairs within the cultural and social environment in which he has grown up, lived and worked. This soon leads to problems, both for the patient and for his partner, particularly in the western world with its increasing complexity, its highly individualistic orientation and its ever looser group and family ties.

Even remembering significant recent events is now affected. The patient may have difficulty in recalling events in which he was personally involved a day or a week before. He also finds it difficult to place his daily experiences in the right order.

Moreover he is often unable to recall memories from the past in the right order. This inability to situate happenings in time is part of a disturbed experience of time. Events are beacons in the current of time. When they disappear from memory or can not be put in the correct order, the experience of time itself undergoes a change and time becomes less determinable.

Disturbed experience of time and space
If the experience of time changes, events and things lose their logical connection. Ties with present, past and future become looser: the patient sometimes gets lost in time. He occasionally gets muddled about which month or year it is.

This disturbed experience of time causes serious difficulties with activities which call for timing and planning, such as the management of one's personal financial affairs or arranging household activities such as well-planned shopping, necessary repairs or cleaning, or arranging a meal with friends or making vacation plans. When the patient goes shopping, he comes home with the wrong purchases. He often fails to have the necessary ingredients in the house, has difficulty in preparing a reasonably varied meal and sometimes misses out meals altogether. The consequence can be a loss of weight and a shortage of fluid and vitamins or anemia. This can have a further detrimental effect on the mental functions.

He is now less capable of keeping his attention selectively directed to a particular thing, which means that he continually loses sight of the goal of his attention and is easily distracted. Time and space are closely connected with one another in the world as we experience it. The patient in the initial stage of dementia is less capable of efficiently organizing and demarcating his personal environment, so that he no longer knows where to find things which he frequently moves from one place to another. He often skips his daily wash, sometimes because he is convinced that he has already done it. But the motive to do so – personal hygiene, looking clean at work, looking well-groomed if you go down town or visit friends – is no longer present. The conception of the value of, and responsibility for personal hygiene only comes at a late stage in human development and with the loss of mental faculties it already disappears early on.

Speech also alters. The change in the patient's world leads to a deterioration in his powers of conversation, to empty words. He has very little to say and his family and friends notice that he has become so silent. Conversely, he may be very talkative at times, but his conversation is often tangential.

His movements express hesitation and he walks as though he is searching for something. He does not exactly know where it was he was going to and his family notice that his movements are becoming slower and more hesitant. This locomotor disturbance is especially noticeable when he is left to himself. If he is stimulated by someone else or if he gets emotional, he is capable of walking quickly. Periodically he is engaged in non-purposeful activity in the form of nervous agitation, fidgeting with his hands and being unable to remain sitting quietly for any length of time.

Emotional reactions

Decreasing attention to his environment and to other people leads to an impoverishment of his emotions. He becomes less expressive, exhibits less varied emotions.

The cognitive and functional level of the Alzheimer patient in this stage drops back to that of an eight-year-old child. His actions are now motivated by what is of immediate concrete concern to him. The future and tomorrow become vague notions. Sometimes that leads to a feeling of carefreeness and indifference, sometimes to fearful expectation; that partly depends on personal aptitude and temperament. By denying or trivializing his diminished cognitive functions and the accompanying problems, the patient defends himself against the impairment of the integrity of his personality, which has been brought about by the disease. If he is then suddenly confronted with it in a particular situation, this can lead to acute panic, totally blocking his power of thought and finding expression in a powerful emotional discharge, such as a violent fit of crying or an outburst of rage. Because the beginning of the decline in his mental functions is almost imperceptible, because he does not feel physically ill, because nobody can tell him what is going on, because he also has days on which he still functions reasonably well, for all these reasons he is able to deny his loss of functionality. He cannot agree with his partner or children, who see it all in a different light, and send him to the doctor. That can lead to distrust and occasionally to delusions of infidelity, with which he tries to explain something which he can no longer reason out logically.

He loses the power of objectivity, of checking his conjectures and notions against reality, which is now slowly beginning to escape him. The experience of this loss, of a world which is slipping away from him, of powerlessness, of feelings of inadequacy sometimes leads to fits of weeping and the complaint: "I wish I were dead." These periodical waves of depression do not usually result in serious thoughts of, or attempts at suicide, but this possibility cannot be entirely excluded. It can on occasion be very difficult to distinguish these depressive episodes, especially when there is also insomnia, a lack of emotional expression, talking less than previously and walking more slowly, from genuine depression. The latter must always be ruled out by means of a psychiatric examination. Depression can be effectively treated and in that case the disturbances of the mental functions, which resulted from the depression, usually disappear after a period of time.

In this stage (stage I) the patient is sometimes still able to camouflage his shortcomings from those with whom he is not in daily contact and he can be friendly and charming. These are sometimes the people he finds willing to lend an ear to his complaints about his partner and caregiver. But if the other person questions him more closely, the patient soon becomes more cautious and retreats. He needs allies who will back him up. Some patients become more and more silent. Others become extremely talkative, often about their past experiences. Their thoughts and actions are self-centred and they are no longer able to judge themselves or other people objectively.

If another person confronts the patient with his inability to perform certain activities or to remember events, he will look for a plausible explanation, which at the same time often functions as an excuse and defense: "I'm getting old, why should it be so abnormal to forget something now and again – that belongs to getting old, doesn't it?" The inclination to be easily irritated may lead to sudden outbursts of rage and shrieking. The patient is cross with himself, because he is aware of his diminished mental faculties. He is cross with the other person, if that person intentionally or unintentionally confronts him with it.

An indefinable feeling of anxiety, the inability to structurize his own time, the vagueness of the future and sometimes the sensation of the faster passing of time, which is accentuated even more as a result of his fears, all this leads to restlessness. He is continually appealing to his partner with questions such as: "When are we going home?" "Where are we going?" "What am I doing here?" "What's the time?". The often compulsive questioning is apparently not so much directed towards getting a particular answer, which he cannot really do anything with anyway. It is more an appeal to the other person. What he is asking is: "What must I do, I want to do something to get rid of the tension, but I cannot do it by myself, help me, put me in touch with my environment again." In a sense it is the verbal equivalent of restlessly wandering to and fro. Taking the patient's mind off himself and engaging him in other purposeful activities is often more effective than answering his questions. If his appeal is ignored, however, he can become infuriated. Sometimes he begins on an activity, which then ends up in aimless repetition of a certain component action thereof, because he no longer knows how to go any further. .

Disturbed sense of reality

Although more common in the stages II and III, disturbances of perception can sometimes lead to hallucinations: seeing persons or things which are not there in reality. It is usually a question of seeing people in the house whom he does not know, or he has seen relatives who died some time ago. Less common is hearing people talk, who are not actually there. This may be augmented by impaired hearing.

The personal feelings towards the other person, especially the partner, are sometimes very unstable and can change from one moment to the next from extreme friendliness to downright hostility. An apparently insignificant gesture or word from the other person can be enough to trigger this off. His mood can then affect his disturbed perception. For instance, during a visit to a doctor, where the daughter was describing the mother's problems, the patient became more and more agitated. She suddenly became furious with her daughter and reproached her with: "How can you say such things, you are not my daughter, you are someone else, you look unfamiliar, I'm frightened of you!" and began to cry uncontrollably. In such a situation there is a vicious circle: a remark or gesture by the partner is immediately interpreted as hostile and personally intended, which stirs up negative and sometimes violent emotion in the patient. The violent emotion influences and colors his already unstable perception, whereby the partner suddenly seems to change his appearance and lose his familiarity for the patient. That in turn reinforces the ever present, indeterminate feeling of fear, which is now directed towards the partner. A state of panic arises, which may be released in the form of a fit of crying, swearing, shouting, running away or even in violence.

As the disease progresses, the emotions and the perception become increasingly unstable and the chance of behavioral disturbances such as agitation becomes ever greater. Under the influence of strong negative emotions the patient's functioning can even stagnate temporarily. Strong emotions diminish the efficiency of his activities and block the mental faculties which are still present. His behavior then soon becomes determined by *fight or flight*. Thus behavioral disturbances can have a detrimental influence on the patient's cognition and functionality. It is very important for the caregiver to be familiar with these disturbances and know why and when they occur. Only in stage IV of the disease, when perception and emotion are almost completely deadened, does the patient become calmer again, even apathetic.

From the above it can be seen that the patient is extremely sensitive about everything which he experiences as a negative judgment of himself. His reactions are colored by the fact that he is inclined to take everything personally. Thus he is always on the defensive. As mentioned earlier, there are individual differences in the occurrence and nature of these symptoms of disturbed behavior. Often one or two of the symptoms are to the fore. Some patients react more intensely than others to the disintegration of their world. Many of the behavioral disturbances discussed above do certainly not always occur in the early stage of the illness. But they sometimes may be the first warning sign of beginning dementia. In the following stages of the disease, when perception becomes increasingly disturbed and insight into ones own situation and the availability of adequate means of expressing oneself are continually decreasing, the chance of serious behavioral disturbances becomes ever greater. Until finally the disease extinguishes virtually all perception and emotion and the patient sinks into almost complete oblivion.

Need of structure

As regular a life as possible with a set daily pattern creates a favorable environment in which to care for the patient. The less tense the caregiver is, the calmer the patient will be. If the caregiver knows beforehand what situations he can expect and how the patient reacts to them, that can contribute considerably to the peace of mind of them both. It is important that the patient's environment and his day and night program are structurized as much as possible. That does not mean that the patient cannot be left alone for a moment. Sometimes he has need of this. The principle of caring for the patient is to stimulate his sense of self-respect as far as possible. The less he has the idea that he is being organized and patronized, the more positive his feelings will be. Thus in this first stage of the illness the patient can still perform most of the routine activities of daily self-care, provided he is tactfully reminded and encouraged by the caregiver. It is better to let him carry out these activities himself as far as possible, even though he does not always do everything to perfection.

Activities which call for insight, judgment, planning and organization, such as dealing with financial affairs or the general organization and overview of the household, have to be taken over from him. Otherwise he can be put at a serious disadvantage. With the recreational activities the goal is to keep the patient functional and occupied as long as possible, in the relaxed atmosphere of a game. These activities should be attuned to the mental faculties which he still has. Some patients can occupy themselves for a considerable length of time, once they have been given a start. Others need continual encouragement and personal attention. However, the caregiver – whether it is the partner or a professional caregiver – must always treat the patient on an equal footing and not act as a pseudo-tutor or surrogate parent. That can sometimes be difficult.

Some patients already need a professional caregiver in this stage. The patient neither chooses nor asks for him. Therefore he does not always accept him in his house. Sometimes the patient views the caregiver as a home help and treats him as such. In such situations the caregiver needs to exercise a great deal of tact. It may sometimes be possible to introduce the caregiver to the patient as a temporary guest. The 'guest' then obligingly offers his help and asks the patient how he wants things done. The patient likes it if the caregiver asks him to help perform an activity together. What he does not want, is to be ordered about.

This first stage of Alzheimer's disease, in which the patient needs continuing help with more complicated activities calling for planning, such as dealing with financial affairs, paying rent and settling accounts, overviewing the housekeeping, planning and making the necessary purchases, lasts for about two years. At the end of this stage the cognitive functions have declined to such an extent that a more intensive form of care than supervision and stimulation alone is required.

What the patient can do himself
√ put his signature on checks, deeds, policies
√ draw money from the bank
√ pay small cash sums, for example for food, cleaning products, candy, newspapers and magazines

Encourage patient to
√ give all bills to the caregiver
√ give all official papers to the caregiver (tax returns etc.)
√ show checks received to caregiver and cash them or deposit them together with him

Intervene supervise and if necessary prevent
√ prevent alterations to documents and subsequent signing of legal documents by patient, such as will, benefactions, conveyance of real estate, termination of marriage settlement, changes in name of executor of will. The patient is unable to oversee the consequences
√ prevent impulsive spending of large sums of money (e.g. gambling in casino, giving to sects or religious denominations)
√ prevent use of credit cards by patient for payment
√ prevent patient from becoming victim of door-to-door salesmen
√ keep an eye on withdrawal of money from bank account, bearing balance in mind
√ keep an eye on writing out of checks (filling in payee and amount) by the patient
√ keep an eye on keeping cash book up to date
√ keep an eye on taking exact amount of money needed for shopping
√ keep an eye on mailing of accounts and payments

Partial take-over
√ enter shopping list in clearly legible writing in notebook and mention what items should cost (in connection with housekeeping budget)

Total take-over

√ determine and supervise total housekeeping budget

√ receive pension payments

√ draw up budget for major expenditure such as: moving house, alterations to house, furniture, a party

√ management of all financial affairs such as: tax returns, rent, instalments, insurance/premiums, gas/water/ electricity/television, send bills from doctors/therapists on to insurance company

√ keep the lawyer informed of the patient's mental condition and refer him to the doctor attending him (the lawyer may personally want to contact the doctor in connection with the question of accountability)

√ appoint official trustee for patient's financial affairs

Attitude towards the patient

√ realize and appreciate that money is important for self-preservation, care for ones own life and a feeling of independence

√ face up to fact that no longer being in control of ones own money represents total dependence on the caregiver and calls for great faith in his honesty

√ see that he always has some money to spend as he wishes

√ compliment him on the way the money is spent or make no comment

√ in the event of financial or legal problems, call in experts

√ always discuss all financial problems with all members of the family to prevent controversy

√ realize that, for the very reason that the patient denies his actual condition, he lacks the insight and judgment to take responsible financial decisions

√ realize that, for the very reason the patient denies his condition, he views above all tactless interference with his financial affairs by another person with suspicion

What the patient can do himself

√ name coins and bills and distinguish the different values
√ cope with numbers from 1 to 100: count with insight – backwards and forwards; have an idea of amounts from 1 to 100 and express them in figures; add and subtract numbers of not more than two figures; multiply and divide two figure numbers by one figure numbers
√ name numbers from 1 to 100, which are called out or written in letters, in separate figures
√ form an idea of the amount which is expressed in numbers from 1 to 100
√ distinguish between less, much and more
√ survey cause and effect; if one spends money, then one has less money left

Remind and encourage patient to

√ pay at the check-out, wait for change and put it in his purse
√ sort the change out at home into bills and coins of equal value and put them into the appropriate compartments in separate cans or boxes
√ count the coins per can
√ figure out the total value of the number of dimes
√ put the coins in a row of ten and piles of five
√ make his own donations, gifts or contributions

Intervene supervise and if necessary prevent

√ ensure that it is only a question of handling money and not of knowing exactly the number of coins or the result of the count
√ the use of a calculator
√ help with counting, reading and writing numbers which requires knowledge of symbols; this ability often remains intact into the beginning of stage III
√ prevent giving him sums which are beyond him
√ prevent demonstratively correcting his errors

Partial take-over

√ continue to involve the patient in financial affairs by discussing them with him in a way he understands

√ keep him used to handling money by letting him save and spend money himself

√ regularly discuss the objective of saving with him by asking questions such as:"What are you going to buy with this money?" or saying: "We have almost enough money to go out for a meal together. That's great!"

√ keep him informed of the amount saved by letting him count the money. For example, put the tin with the quarters in front of him and say: "Count up how many cents we already have. Put them in rows so that I can look as well."

√ decide together with the patient when the money is going to be spent and let him pay himself

Total take-over

√ keep the patient constructively involved with money

√ collect six transparent food boxes with mouths wide enough to get your hand in easily to keep the different coins in

√ keep the patient involved in writing out checks and paying bills

Attitude

√ realize that, even if the patient no longer knows the economic value of money, it nevertheless still keeps its significance for him as such:

. the realization that money is necessary to support oneself is usually retained up to the end of stage II

. the patient's frequently voiced reproach: "They are taking my money away from me" does not necessarily imply an accusation against another person; the illusion that his money is taken away from him can result from the way he experiences the loss of mental faculties

. money can become a symbol of all his losses

. holding someone responsible for his loss is a way of explaining the loss and an attempt to get a grip on the situation

. by hiding what threatens to be taken away from him, he can defend himself

What the patient can do himself
- √ turn on ignition and start the engine
- √ press on the accelerator and accelerate
- √ apply the breaks
- √ shift gears
- √ drive on quiet streets and roads
- √ turn off ignition
- √ park the car
- √ fill the gas tank

Remind and encourage patient to
- √ patient should definitely be discouraged even in this early stage from driving a car, in particular when by himself. On quiet, familiar streets and roads he may be able to manage on his own

Partial take-over
- √ check gas and oil
- √ make sure that the ignition key is removed before leaving the car
- √ lock the car door
- √ remember the location where the car is parked

Total take-over
- √ driving on busy streets and roads
- √ general maintenance of the car
- √ obtaining new driver's licence and car registration
- √ car insurance

Attitude
- √ although driving skills vary considerably in this stage, the majority of patients is unable to handle emergencies and unexpected situations. Panic can easily occur with disastrous consequences. Most patients can be convinced to stop driving when presented with a reason; some patients accept the caregiver's concern for their memory loss, other patients may be convinced that there are physical problems or medications which make driving hazardous. They will usually accept an order from the doctor not to drive. Some states in the US have passed laws that persons with Alzheimer's disease be reported to the Department of Motor Vehicles

What the patient can do himself	√ open the front door after hearing the doorbell and let the guest(s) in √ pour out a drink √ make simple snacks √ pass round, present things from a tray √ empty ashtray √ lay table (for maximum four people), put out plates, glasses, cutlery and table napkins √ go with guest to front door and open and shut it √ see also STAGE I THE KITCHEN
Remind and encourage	√ the beginning of each of these activities
Intervene supervise and if necessary prevent	√ the patient getting stuck in the action:complying with a request such as: "Take that glass to the kitchen" is a complex task, which can no longer be performed at the end of stage I since a task like this consists of: . understanding spoken language . connecting language with object (the glass) . connecting action asked for with the glass . a. look at the glass; b. pick up the glass; c. know where the kitchen is (orientation), know how to go to the kitchen and put it down there – any of these components may be disturbed
Partial take-over	√ see to extra things such as decorations, lighted candles, enough chairs √ make sure the patient gets enough attention and is treated as equal partner in the conversation √ help to keep the conversation simple √ see that the conversation between patient and a guest is not interrupted and avoid having two people talking to him at the same time √ during the conversation help him to continue his story

Total
take-over
√ the general organization and preparation
√ take cork out of, or cap off bottle
√ light candles

Attitude
√ let the patient welcome the guests who come to visit him
√ give him tasks before, during and after the visit
√ inform the visitors beforehand of the patient's handicap
√ compliment the patient

What the patient can do himself	√ pick up the phone and carry on a conversation with someone he knows √ call someone to the phone √ phone people he knows if the phone numbers are on a clear list in a set place √ order things by phone with the aid of a shopping list
Remind and encourage patient to	√ phone children, family and friends √ write down name and phone number of people who have rung up
Partial take-over	√ help him look up numbers in phone directory √ if necessary write down phone number and place beside phone √ look out for merchandizing by phone
Total take-over	√ write down names and phone numbers in large letters and figures and put somewhere clearly visible in a fixed position √ compile a list with names and phone numbers of the family for emergency use and attach this list to the phone √ check telephone bill
Attitude	√ let him pick up the phone if he wants to do so √ take tactful action if repeated calls are made to same person, who finds this tiresome √ take account of the fact that the patient can no longer remember, pass on or write down phone messages

What the   √ prepare and put out feeding bowl with ready-to
patient can   eat feed, seed or water
do himself   √ feed fish
                    √ clean out hutch, doghouse, cage, aquarium
                    √ take the dog out

Remind and   √ clean feeding bowl every day
encourage   √ take the dog out at a time arranged beforehand
patient to   √ feed pets at set times
if necessary   √ give the dog extra water after exertion
explain

Intervene   √ determine right sort and amount of feed for all
supervise if   pets
necessary   √ remove undesirable smells
                    √ look after sick animals

Partial   √ remove animal hairs
take-over   √ inspect for and remove fleas and ticks

Total   √ accept ultimate responsibility for all his pets;
take-over   for example:
                        . see that pets do not run or fly away
                        . put on a flea collar
                        . cut nails
                        . consult vet if animal is sick

Attitude   √ respect his love of his pet
                    √ if necessary partially take on care of his pets without
                        patient noticing

What the patient can do himself	√ mow the grass with a hand mower √ cut the hedge with hand shears which can be used with one hand √ plant bulbs, plants and shrubs √ weed and rake √ push a wheelbarrow √ shovel in and out √ dig holes √ put waste in bags and remove √ determine when something is ready to be gathered, picked or consumed √ distinguish between sound and damaged fruit √ recognize and remove withered parts of flowers and/or vegetables √ water with hosepipe and watering can √ paint the fence
Encourage patient to if necessary explain step by step	√ begin and complete all separate actions √ clear away tools/materials used and remove waste
Intervene supervise if necessary	√ determine amount of water for spraying √ distribution of shrubs and bulbs when planting √ determine depth in digging holes
Partial take-over	√ if necessary give patient the tools he needs √ take over the finishing touch, e.g. cutting the edges of a lawn √ determine time for planting and pruning
Total take-over	√ sowing seeds √ spreading fertilizer and using weed killer
Attitude	√ show appreciation of his work √ let him work in his own way √ if necessary intervene as casually as possible

What the patient can do himself	√ play cards as formerly but in a slower tempo (e.g. no longer participate in a bridge drive) √ read newspapers and magazines √ play a musical instrument √ handicrafts using a simple, familiar pattern √ knitting, crochet, embroidery √ keep collections up to date, e.g. photos and stamps √ paint, draw, clay modeling √ do jigsaw puzzles √ go for walks, cycle, go fishing (rod and line) √ gymnastics √ (folk) dancing √ sports, such as pool, bowling, swimming, golf
Remind and encourage patient to	√ take plenty of physical exericse, preferably out of doors √ go on with his hobbies √ go to his own club or association
Intervene observe and if necess- ary prevent	√ continually stimulate him to undertake activities and stimulate and guide his remaining initiative and his concentration so that he does not drift away from what he is doing √ prevent distracting, disturbing stimuli from the environment √ see that he wears glasses and has a hearing aid if necessary
Partial take-over	√ put necessary materials out ready √ accompany him on cycle rides; visits to museums; to performances such as concerts, opera, musicals etc.; on walks √ accompany him to clubs for recreational and hobby activities with a group √ do a concentration game with him, e.g. Mikado: 26 colored sticks are mixed up in a pile or in a row packed closely together; the players have to pick up a stick each time with a hook without moving the others √ join with the patient in singing, making music, dancing, swimming etc.

**Total
take-over**

√ planning vacations
√ find out which of his senses and which functions are
the best developed and make use of this, eg: counting
up, conversation, humor, manual skill, music and
dance, sports & games

Attitude

√ do not urge the patient to undertake activities if he is
not familiar with them or does not enjoy them
√ regularly do recreational activities with him; realize that
he himself lacks the initiative, the concentration or the
motivation to perform structurized activities
√ emphasize doing things together and experiencing
activities together, being involved in something, not
having to be on his own in an increasingly confusing
world
√ use the shared experiences as a topic of conversation
√ the patient must be given every opportunity to express
his experiences in words or gestures
√ if people listen to him attentively, he feels important
and safe again
√ if he has difficulty in expressing what he is
experiencing, he must be helped
√ experiences which cannot be shared make for a lonely
world; this applies both to the patient and to the
caregiver

What the patient can do himself	√ use most words in the daily spoken language √ put the emphasis correctly on the right part of the word (through difference in pitch, strength, duration) √ be guided by concrete causal thinking √ follow his own train of thought √ follow someone else's train of thought if it is sufficiently concrete
Remind and encourage patient to	√ play the broken word connection game. The partner/caregiver shows a card with part of a word and asks the patient to add another part of a word to it, so as to make a compound word eg: candle – light √ choose words from the game
Intervene observe and if necessary prevent	√ towards the end of stage I it is no longer possible to make causal connections. For instance: *soapsuds*: the patient no longer knows that the suds are the result of the contact of soap with water. Or *breadcrumb*: that the crumbs are the result of crumbling the bread. √ the patient can still use compound words, in which one part is a further description of the other part, until the middle of stage II
Partial take-over	√ do the broken word connection game together, whereby a spontaneous conversation can start up √ answer his questions in a sensible, understandable, concrete way in proper sentences; answer in such a way that it sets him thinking and he asks further questions √ if necessary help him to find compound words by giving him the first part √ give a maximum of two choices for the first part of the compound word; offer a maximum of four choices for the second part

**Total
take-over**

√ for use in the game collect words which are com-
posed of cause and effect connections, such as:
thunder-bolt, left-over, cat-call, candle-light, wind-
blown, soap-suds, bees-wax, bed-sore, water-fall,
chicken-pox, pig-skin, bread-crumb

√ collect compound words, where one part is the further
description of the other part:, rain-coat, door-mat, pen-
knife, tea-cup, head-ache, bee-hive, arm-chair, snow-
ball, wash-tub, fire-place, video-tape, dog-house

√ write parts of words in large block letters on paper,
then cut them out and paste onto stiff cards

Attitude

√ provide the possibility of the patient keeping his use of
language as long as possible by letting him live and
work with words

√ realize that the loss of the connection between cause
and effect is accompanied by the loss of logical
thinking

√ things he can no longer explain and understand make
him frightened and unsure of himself

√ the patient must get the feeling that he can rely on the
other person, his caregiver, to pilot him through the
now so confusing world

√ do not ask questions which begin with: why, what for,
what with (these emphasize cause and effect)

What the patient can do himself

√ orientate himself in his own home
√ carry out the following actions:
√ . vacuum clean . dust . make bed . change bed
. clean toilet . clean refrigerator . sweep and swab down
. clean windows . clean car .polish silver and brass
. clean shoes
. put garbage can outside
. put flowers in a vase
. wash up, dry up and put away
. do the hand-wash (not washing machine)
. hang the washing up with clothespins
. fold up the washing and put things on coat hangers
. take clothes to dry cleaners in the neighbourhood
. use a spray can
. adjust faucets for the right water temperature
. fill bucket to desired level
. know where cleaning products are kept
. distinguish between some of the familiar cleaning products
. have an idea of the quantities needed
. use the cleaning product in the proper fashion
. use sandpaper
. knock a nail in or pull it out

Remind and encourage patient to
if necessary
explain
step by step

√ begin on and complete activities
√ wear glasses and hearing aid whilst working
√ wear shoes instead of slippers or mules (in connection with slipping and falling)
√ only dust or clean at eye level in case of dizziness
√ give flowers fresh water
√ properly clean forks with remains of food
√ regularly put out clean washing up cloths, dishtowels, hand towels and dusters
√ rinse out sponge and chamois leather
√ clean inside of buckets

Intervene
supervise,
assist and
if necessary
prevent

√ physical incapability of performing the activity
√ standing on a ladder or chair
√ overtiredness; inclination to fall
√ wet or slippery floors
√ use of sharp objects
√ proper use of cleansing agents and choice of right amount
√ proper use of disinfectants such as bleach (keep an eye on the concentration)
√ distinguishing between white and colored wash
√ careful rinsing to get rid of soapsuds
√ proper use of hammer, pincers, axe, scissors

**Partial
take-over**

√ decide on what cleaning activities to do on which which day
√ tidy up the room before the patient starts to clean
√ cleaning of valuable, breakable and delicate objects
√ help the patient when he loses the overall picture in performing an activity, such as rinsing thoroughly after a hand wash or folding up the wash
√ before use by the patient check the contents of the spray can as given on the label
√ put the materials and objects needed for an activity out ready
√ maintenance of furniture, carpet and floors

**Total
take-over**

√ put away breakable objects
√ see that the house is adequately lit
√ see that windows on the top storey are always closed
√ shut all windows out of precaution if patient is alone (only transoms open or windows with window guards)
√ arrange the furniture so that the patient has enough room in which to move about (to prevent him from losing his balance)
√ stick reflecting stickers on sharp corners and fittings
√ remove poisonous indoor plants
√ remove all spray cans with dangerous substances
√ remove all inflammable, caustic or toxic cleaning products

Total take-over

√ put away all substances which are dangerous if swallowed, or in contact with the eyes and skin
√ clean windows
√ do the ironing
√ lower the temperature of the boiler
√ replace or remove rugs with raised edges and rugs which slide easily or steady them with nonslip devices
√ see that shelves in cupboards are firmly secured and remove heavy objects from top shelves
√ make cupboards emptier and more surveyable; remove unnecessary objects and leave remainder in set places
√ remove thresholds or paint the corners in a striking color
√ stairs with two banisters
√ safety device for power points (sockets)
√ throw away all old medicines and lock away medicines to be used. Most patients do not know what medicines they take or what they were prescribed for
√ supervise all household activities
√ keep the house as tidy and orderly as possible
√ always put all objects back in the place familiar to the patient
√ prevent alterations in arrangement of the furniture (pieces of furniture are orientation points for the patient)

Attitude

√ do not leave the patient alone when he/she is agitated
√ show you take account of:
  . his need of independence and a critical attitude
  . his limited knowledge of words . his sensitivity to graphic things and events, cosiness and cheerfulness or quarrels
  . his difficulty in seeing cause and effect
  . his inability to picture a situation clearly
  . his lack of self-confidence
√ unobtrusively relieve him of work which requires too much or too stressful physical and mental exertion

What the patient can do himself	√ go to a local shop unaccompanied √ cross the road(sometimes he may be hesitant) √ go shopping with the aid of a shopping list (up to three articles) √ recognize a product previously used by color and form of the packing √ make his own choice of bread, cold cuts etc. by pointing to them when he cannot remember them by name √ ask where he can find a particular article √ take desired article out of the rack, place in shopping cart and put on the counter √ get out money and give to the cashier (but patient often no longer knows what things cost and how much change he should have)
Remind and encourage patient to	√ go to the shop to buy what he needs √ consult shopping list √ ask for change at the cash desk
Intervene supervise and prevent	√ do shopping alone where public transport is necessary √ impulsive spending of money on daily necessities
Partial take-over	√ draw up shopping list together: articles, amounts weight, color, numbers; done so that shop assistant can help if necessary √ give patient shopping list and shopping bag √ help him choose when buying clothes and shoes
Total take-over	√ have an identity disc made (chain or bracelet) and see that it is worn √ estimate how much money the patient needs for the shopping and do not give much more than the amount required √ hang up a list of things to be bought
Attitude	√ do not reproach the patient if he comes back with the wrong articles and/or comes 'too late'

What the patient can do himself

√ perform simple and familiar actions, such as passing things, turning the faucet on and off, opening pots and bottles, stir, peel, cut, clean vegetables, wash his hands, put things away, pour out, knead, throw things away, put things in a row/pile, serve out, fold up, toast bread, squeeze, rinse, wash out etc.

√ make tea and coffee in his own familiar way

√ hand over familiar kitchen utensils

√ turn on/off gas or electric cooker

√ see when something is boiling

√ mix up ingredients

√ find something to satisfy his hunger and quench his thirst

Remind and encourage patient to

√ begin on kitchen activities

√ carefully wash prepared potatoes and vegetables

Intervene supervise

√ use of seasoning or relish for food, butter or oil

√ turning on and off of gas flame or hotplate

√ keep an eye on cooking time, boiling over, boiling dry and burning on

√ clear up (used or dirty) implements between times

√ conservation of food and drink and judge reliability

Partial take-over

√ menu for breakfast and lunch

√ determine time of meals

√ choose time to start preparing meal

Total
take-over

√ retain the ultimate responsibility for the household
√ draw up menu for hot meal
√ take charge of matches
√ check whether food is fully cooked or not
√ pour off cooking water
√ pour out or ladle out hot gravy
√ reduce seasoning to salt, pepper and a few herbs (two)
√ replace large, heavy pans by small, lightweight pans
√ clear out overfull kitchen cupboards as far as possible
   (enough items for two people), but leave the remaining
   items as far as possible in the same place
√ check whether cooker has been turned off after cooking
√ do not set water heaters too high so as to avoid burns

Attitude

√ encourage and praise the patient in all his efforts by
   means of gestures, mime and inflection of voice
√ avoid demonstrative corrective actions in the presence
   of the patient, e.g. further work on potatoes peeled by
   him/her, where the peel has not been totally removed
√ accept the fact that the patient cannot always work
   purposefully and efficiently
√ continue to involve the patient in kitchen activities
   even if his performance is not always a success
√ when there are various choices for the patient, choose
   the most functional
√ take into account that the patient can no longer form
   an idea of a complicated action

What the patient can do himself	√ recognize the external parts of the body, name them indicate them on himself and another person √ indicate functions of nose (smell), ears (hear), eyes (see), mouth (speak, eat) and lips (kiss, talk) √ know what you do with your arms (wave, bend,lift) hands (grasp/pinch, caress/give a smack), legs and feet (stand, walk) √ distinguish, indicate and name: left-right, above-below and in front-behind
Remind and encourage patient to	√ name and point to parts of body whilst bathing (together) and dressing (casually); for example: "Will you show me your hands?" or "Will you wash my back?"
Partial take-over	√ body scheme exercises: √ name parts of body and let the patient point to them on his own body or someone else's; point to parts of body and let the patient name them √ exercise with body figure puzzle (see 'total take-over') . at the front and back of the figure, point to and name or let the patient point to and name parts of the body . let him take the parts out one by one by saying: "Give me the right leg." (In this stage (I) the patient can still look at the mirror image) . independently or after being given them, put the pieces of the disassembled puzzle together again . do this exercise together daily before bathing √ ask about simple bodily functions, such as: "What do you do with your nose?"
Total take-over	√ the composition of the body figure puzzle: 1 make two figures of an adult man or woman seen from the front and the back, with the parts of the body clearly discernible 2 stick the figures onto plywood or sturdy cardboard and then saw or cut out the separate parts of the body 3 it is advisable to enclose the human figure in a frame (shifting of parts is confusing)

Attitude   √ realize that at the end of stage I the *conscious* certainty
of the patient towards his own body scheme may begin
to blur

√ realize that, in view of the activities of daily life (ADL),
it is important to maintain the awareness of the body
scheme as long as possible

What the patient can do himself

√ orientate himself in his own bathroom
√ wash himself at the lavatory basin
√ perform the separate actions of showering/bathing in the right order (see under Encourage)

Remind and encourage patient to

√ put dressing gown/housecoat out ready
√ not to lock the door
√ begin to shower, bath or wash at the lavatory basin
√ perform the actions as far as possible sitting down and making use of the handgrasps fixed to the wall
√ wash the whole of his body
√ use soap and shampoo
√ wash the back with a back brush
√ carefully rinse off soap and thoroughly dry himself, especially between the folds of the skin
√ rub his whole body with a moisturizer
√ use a deodorant in the armpits when needed
√ hang the towel up to dry
√ remove dirty linen to the linen bin

Intervene observe for and if necessary prevent

√ expressions of feelings of discomfort which may indicate giddiness, for example: wobbling; holding onto something; putting his hands in front of his eyes; looking frightened; looking white-faced; saying: "Wait a minute!"; mentioning a feeling of nausea
√ itching and scratching himself which may be caused by using too much soap; not rinsing the soap off thoroughly; use of certain medicines; anemia; (pubic) lice, fleas, scabies
√ body odor, unwashed parts of the body, dirty nails
√ look out for bath running over
√ abnormalities of the skin such as being dry, chafed, taut; swelling (edema); redness; paleness; damage; too hot or too cold skin; fungus infections; rash such as caused by medication; blisters; wounds; boils or other local inflammation of the skin; bruises which may indicate a fall; lumps

Partial take-over

√ stick nonslip material in shower/bath and in front of wash bowl
√ put stool or chair in shower or in front of wash bowl
√ see that bathroom is at right temperature
√ put out towel and toilet requisites
√ put noxious substances out of reach
√ make sure bathroom door cannot be locked
√ when patient is no longer able to: wash his back and feet

Total take-over

√ consult doctor in event of a fall, serious feelings of discomfort and skin abnormalities
√ take responsibility for optimum hygiene
√ put on ointment, bandaid, etc., give prescribed medication, disinfect cuts and wounds, look after infected areas
√ avoid use of hot water bottle or electric blanket during sleep
√ if necessary warm bed beforehand and use flannel sheets
√ regulate temperature of hot water as well as possible
√ clearly mark hot water faucet (red sticker)
√ buy skin care products (non-alkaline) and soft toilet paper, to prevent infections in anal cleft
√ check whether shower/bath faucets are turned off after use
√ check whether bath water has run away
√ to be recommended:
  . purchase supporting foam rubber mattress with big compartments (variable pressure on skin)
  . buy high-protein food (monthly renewal of skin cells takes about twenty percent of the daily need of protein)

Attitude

√ take account of the patient's cultural background, philosophy of life and previous history
√ make it clear that prevention is better than cure
√ take account of the patient's needs and habits; tempo; pain, itching etc.; privacy; what should/should not be repeated to others; feelings of shame
√ avoid confrontation, avoid grabbing the patient suddenly

What the patient can do himself	√ perform fine finger movements √ shorten fingernails by means of cutting and/or filing √ polish nails √ wash hands, dry them and rub in skin cream √ point to left and right hand, on himself and on another person √ name the fingers and thumb
Remind and encourage patient to explain	√ perform fine finger movements every day, e.g. writing; drawing; clay modeling; sticking in stamps and photos; knitting; crocheting √ clean finger nails
Intervene observe for and if necessary prevent	√ dirty hands and nails;sharp nails;frayed cuticles inflamed cuticles; chapped hands; cuts; rash √ negligence in washing hands before and after the meal; after dirty work; after going to the toilet √ omission of rubbing cream into hands mornings and evenings
Partial take-over	√ put out articles for care of nails and hands √ do additional nail cutting or filing √ keep cuticles trimmed
Total take-over	√ regularly massage fingers one by one and at the same time let the fingers make stretching movements √ purchase of hand care products
Attitude	√ realize the importance of and see to it that hands and nails are well manicured √ be aware that contractures (malformation) of fingers, hands and wrists can arise and take account of this in order to prevent excess loss of function √ realize that continuing to perform hand movements is most important for the patient's functioning √ respect wishes of the patient (or family) as long as they are in conformity with hygiene and safety e.g. with regard to length of nails or polishing nails

What the patient can do himself	√ put on and take off shoes √ wash and dry his feet √ mention pain and indicate the painful spot if requested
Remind and encourage patient to	√ wash feet daily and dry well, particularly between the toes √ put on clean stockings, panty hose or socks every day √ smooth out wrinkles when pulling stockings, panty hose or socks over foot
Intervene observe for and if necessary prevent	√ difficulties with walking √ swollen ankles (edema); chilblains, cold feet; cramp √ too long or blue nails; 'chalk' nails; ingrowing nails √ unequal wearing down of heels of shoes √ holes in shoes, tights, socks √ blisters; sore places between the toes; bunions under big toe, ball of the foot or edge of heel; corns; eczema
Partial take-over	√ put out items for foot care such as foot-bath with water; if necessary an appliance for foot massage √ if necessary dry between the toes √ daily manual check of inside of shoes for unevenness
Total take-over	√ keep toenails short, cut off straight, round off corners √ if necessary arrange for visit to podiatrist for foot care √ where necessary apply ointment, powder and bandaids √ regularly massage the feet and toes with moisturizing cream on top and underneath for at least five minutes (stimulates blood circulation) √ buy comfortable shoes in good time; lightweight, leather, with anti-slip sole and heel √ consult doctor or podiatrist in the event of serious pain or foot injuries
Attitude	√ realize the importance of and see to painless feet and suitable footwear to prevent problems √ be aware that being able to move about independently is of great importance for the patient

What the patient can do himself

√ use his own toothbrush
√ put toothpaste onto toothbrush
√ clean his teeth in the familiar way
√ rinse his mouth
√ rinse off the brush
√ put his dentures into his mouth and take them out
√ clean his dentures and mouth
√ indicate toothache or other oral discomfort
√ on request: show what or where the discomfort is; breathe deeply in and out; open and shut mouth; keep mouth open; stick out tongue; swallow; bite hard; chew; suck; spit out; blow

Remind and encourage patient to
if necessary
explain

√ brush teeth or clean dentures (twice a day)
√ rinse mouth with mouthwash if breath is bad
√ carefully rinse off toothbrush and put it back in the right place
√ if patient has dentures to take them out before going to sleep and put into glass or container
√ use moisturizing cream on the lips
√ spit out mucus into receptacle

Intervene
observe for
and if necess-
ary prevent

√ remains of food between the teeth
√ dirty corners of the mouth
√ dry or scabbed lips
√ badly fitting dentures
√ grinding teeth; this causes earache and damaged molars; certain drugs may increase tooth grinding
√ inflamed gums or mucous membrane

Partial take-over

√ put out requisites for oral and dental care
√ prevent drying out of mucous membrane by:
  . providing three pints of fluid per day
  . keeping air moist in patient's environment
  . checking on side-effects of medicines, such as diuretics, sedatives and neuroleptics (tranquilizers)
  . encouraging rinsing the mouth, three times a day
√ see to it that patient's breath is fresh by
  . giving mint tea after the meal
  . encourage regular meal times etc.

Total take-over

√ make appointments with dentist to prevent dental and digestive problems (at least twice a year), in stage I the patient can still cooperate with the dentist; in later stages this becomes increasingly more difficult if not impossible
√ purchase proper requisites for oral care, including four times a year a soft nylon toothbrush with a sturdy handle

Attitude

√ realize that the mouth is an important means of expression and communication
√ provide the opportunity of cleaning teeth three times a day
√ realize the importance of good oral and dental care for health in general and for digestion in particular and act accordingly

What the patient can do himself

√ recognize his reflection in the mirror
√ wash and dry his/her hair, face, neck and ears
√ apply soap, cream and lipstick
√ take out of own bathroom cupboard: comb, brush, shaver, soap, skin care products, shampoo
√ comb/brush hair
√ shave himself in the familiar way
√ go to the local hairdresser/beautician/barber
√ blow his/her nose

Remind and encourage patient to if necessary explain

√ take toilet requisites out of the cupboard
√ rub cosmetics into the skin
√ wash hands after rubbing in colored cream or powder
√ clean facial skin at end of day and rub in cream
√ wash hair, at least once a week
√ comb and part hair
√ shave
√ go to the hairdresser and, if accustomed, to the beautician

Intervene supervise and if necessary prevent

√ use of the right amount of cosmetics, protective creams etc.
√ smooth, uniform application of cream, powder, lipstick
√ frequent scratching of the head, caused for instance by too dry skin or lice
√ brush/comb hair in style
√ clean ears, eyes, nose and neck
√ skin damage resulting from shaving
√ eczema patches by nostrils, in the auditory duct and behind the ears
√ red-veined or inflamed eyes
√ chapped lips
√ blocked sebaceous glands

Partial take-over

√ comb out tangled hair (beginning at ends, continuing in direction of scalp, in order to avoid pulling out hair)
√ putting up long hair in the desired style
√ clean shaver and regularly disinfect with alcohol
√ replace articles and equipment used to their fixed place

Total take-over

√ arrange patient's daily requisites in bathroom cupboard in an orderly manner so that he can easily find them
√ for women: remove long hairs on chin or upper lip with tweezers if necessary
√ see to ears, eyes and nose, e.g. clean, apply ointment, drops
√ for men trim moustache or beard and trim off protruding hairs from ears and nose
√ purchase shampoo which does not irritate eyes; safety-razor blades and shaving cream; cosmetics
√ consult doctor in the event of abnormalities of skin, ears, eyes, nose
√ accompany patient to hairdresser and/or beautician

Attitude

√ give the patient sincere compliments on his/her appearance
√ only cut long hair short or shave off moustache or beard after consultation with and permission from patient and family
√ ask what the patient usually does with regard to facial skin care, make-up, head and body hair and see that these habits are continued
√ see to it that women do not have hair removed from chin and upper lip with a shaver (after shaving the downy hairs change into bristly hairs)
√ express recognition of the fact that the patient has a pleasantly well-kept appearance; it is his 'visiting card'

What the
patient can
do himself

√ form an idea about what is involved in dressing as a
   sequence of activities
√ choose from not more than five items of outerwear,
   underwear and jewellery
√ choose clothing suited to the season or the weather
√ decide what he/she will or will not wear
√ collect and lay out matching outer- and underwear,
   shoes and jewellery
√ hang up garment on coathanger
√ distinguish between right/left, top/bottom, front/back
√ put on all garments himself
√ carry out all habitual dressing actions: .pick up garment
   and hold it in the right relation to the body
   . adjust body posture to alteration in form of garment
     whilst putting it on
   . pull the garment right on over the joint
   . put head, hands or feet through the appropriate
     opening
   . use a variety of fastenings: buttons, zippers, bows,
     snap fasteners, velcro, hooks and eyes
   . put clothes on tidily
√ indicate when clothes chafe, are too tight, tickle
√ put on watch, bracelet, necklace, earrings

Remind and
encourage
patient to
if necessary
explain
step by step

√ get dressed in the morning
√ begin to dress and undress in the morning and evening
√ dress for special occasions
√ put on clean clothes, e.g. after working in the garden
√ dress in front of the mirror
√ dress and undress sitting down
√ do up and smooth out clothing
√ clean or polish shoes

Intervene
observe for
and if neces-
ary prevent

√ wrong combination of clothes; lack of variation
√ carelessly worn clothes: wrinkles and pleats in tights and
   sleeves; fastenings done up wrong; underskirt showing
√ indecisiveness in choosing clothes
√ fatigue, tightness of the chest, wobbling or tendency to
   fall whilst dressing and undressing

Partial take-over

√ put out chair and stool of about 20 cm in height to put feet on whilst dressing and undressing
√ open and close (intricate) fastenings
√ check clothes for spots, tears, state of fastenings etc.
√ if necessary:
. do up shoelaces
. put belt through loops of trousers or skirt
. knot tie
√ fasten suspenders
√ provide clothing to cover skin in fierce sun

Total take-over

√ limit the clothes in the patient's cupboard to five or less of each item of clothing
√ take photographs of cominations of clothes in the style the patient is used to, hang these photos on inside of cabinet door or stick into album and put this in a clearly visible place; these pictures are a help to the caregiver; he thus knows the patient's preferences as regards clothing and it makes it easier for him to detect initial difficulties in choosing matching clothing
√ repair clothes
√ remove spots/stains
√ decide on purchase of new clothes and look out for: sufficiently broad back; wide armholes; easy fastenings; moisture absorption capacity; clear distinction between front and back; clothes the patient is used to, e.g. not a bra with a front fastening if patient is used to a back fastening; avoid big divergence from style of clothes patient is used to

Attitude

√ allow the patient plenty of time to dress
√ let him do as much as he can himself
√ be present in the background
√ give him sincere compliments on his clothes
√ casually take over actions which confuse the patient
√ avoid taking hold of the patient unexpectedly or roughly (this arouses resistance)

What the patient can do himself

√ lay the table for two people
√ clear the table taking one thing at a time in both hands
√ put vase of flowers and serving dishes on the table
√ take account of table-companions
√ continue acquired table manners
√ serve himself during the meal
√ pass a dish during the meal
√ use table napkin to wipe off mouth, chin, fingers
√ cut food into small pieces with a knife
√ eat and drink without making a mess
√ chew thoroughly
√ whilst chewing notice something inedible and take it out of the mouth
√ finish each mouthful completely
√ move and pick up food with a fork
√ dish out and dish up food with a spoon
√ drink out of a cup, mug, glass
√ suck liquid through a straw
√ put food into the mouth with the fingers
√ lick up something with the tongue
√ take something to eat or drink if hungry or thirsty

Remind and encourage patient to

√ wear the necessary glasses, hearing aid and dentures during the meal
√ perform all necessary actions described above when necessary
√ drink at least three pints of liquid a day

Intervene observe for and prevent

√ taking too hot or too cold food
√ choking

Partial take-over

√ let him eat with his own familiar (solid) cutlery
√ in a restaurant read out the menu and help in making a choice

**Total
take-over**

√ see that there is food which guarantees the
  daily need of carbohydrates, fats, proteins, vitamins and
  minerals
√ vary the menus for the meals
√ eat three times a day at set times
√ be responsible for a comforable room temperature
√ see that the food is served at the right temperature
√ take the patient out to a restaurant
√ look after use of medicines:
  . supervise taking of prescribed medicines
  . at the time indicated hand the patient the medicine
    and also give him a glass of water
  . tell the patient exactly how to take the medicine
  . see that the medicine has been swallowed
  . consult the doctor if there are problems with
    swallowing medicines

Attitude

√ take account of particular eating habits and cultural
  background and act accordingly
√ allow time to say grace before and after meals
√ if necessary unobtrusively fetch something which has
  been 'forgotten', e.g. in laying the table
√ treat the patient in a friendly manner
√ continually involve the patient in the table
  conversation
√ take dishes and plates off the tray before starting to eat
√ if necessary give a clean table napkin
√ allow plenty of time to eat
√ prevent medicines being mixed through a whole
  portion of food or drink

What the patient can do himself

√ go to the toilet if he feels the urge
√ put on light in toilet, shut and lock door, (see Encourage to)
√ adjust his clothes
√ (for men) urinate standing up, direct the urine flow
√ sit down on the toilet and stand up again
√ clean anus and genitals
√ use toilet paper and subsequently put into toilet bowl
√ flush the toilet (if familiar with the flushing system)
√ after going to the toilet, put his clothes in order again
√ unlock and open the door again, put out light, leave toilet and shut the door
√ indicate symptoms of pain, itching and discharge
√ avoid escape of flatus in presence of others

Remind and encourage patient to
if necessary
explain
step by step

√ not to lock toilet door when using the toilet
√ wash hands after going to the toilet
√ in the event of hard motions or constipation:
. begin the day by eating wholemeal bread and yogurt and drinking coffee (no strong tea)
. chew food well, eat slowly and regularly drink a glass of water or other fluid
. going to the toilet regularly: shortly after breakfast sit on the toilet for about ten minutes. (Intake of food stimulates the reflex action of the colon). Preferably with feet on a stool (20 cm high) for better sitting posture
. not to press too long or too hard, this can cause hemorrhoids, fainting or rarely even cerebral hemorrhage
√ wipe off anus carefully in the event of hemorrhoids
√ clean anus with water and apply ointment to anal cleft in event of irritation from hemorrhoids or pain caused by sores
√ urinate before leaving the house for a longer period
√ outside his own house inspect the toilet and toilet seat before use

Intervene
observe and
if necessary
prevent

√ getting lost on the way to the toilet owing to disturbed orientation

√ change in frequency of going to toilet

√ increased urge to urinate or defecate when taking diuretics or laxatives . see that the patient goes to the toilet in time . look out for consequences of too great loss of fluid and salt on account of diuretics and laxatives, such as: occurrence of general muscular weakness, increasing bewilderment, drowsiness, staggering, inclination to fall, knees giving way, nausea, fainting, dry mouth difficulties in swallowing

√ occurrence of decreased urination on account of inability to empty bladder properly, resulting from prostate enlargement or certain medicines such as antidepressants and antipsychotic drugs

√ occurrence of constipation or diarrhea

√ suppression of urge to defecate as result of hard motion or pain in the anus or hemorrhoids

√ complaints about pain or difficulties when urinating or defecating: inspect urine and feces for abnormal color, smell, amount, blood in urine or feces

√ symptoms of bad appetite resulting from constipation such as: feeling full, nausea, gastric acidity, bad breath, restless nights on account of urge to urinate

√ smelling of urine and/or feces

√ re-arranging clothes after visit to toilet

√ urine stains on toes of shoes

√ clean hands and nails

√ dirty toilet seat and floor in front of toilet bowl

√ ease of access to toilet both day and night

√ accessibility of the caregiver

Partial
take-over

In own home:

√ hang up/put out toilet paper, soap, hand towel

√ prevent hard motions and constipation by promoting:
  . adequate physical exercise
  . providing large glass of (lukewarm) water or other liquid directly after getting out of bed in the morning
  . see that the patient gets sufficient fluids by drinking three pints of fluids per day. This avoids thickening and hardening of motions
  . regular meals
  . diet containing sufficient fat and fibers

√ in the event of constipation massage above the buttocks and abdomen from the right-hand groin region via the upper abdomen to the left-hand groin region

Outside his own home:

√ check:
  . quick and easy access to toilet and if necessary accompany patient to toilet door
  . good light on the way to the toilet and absence of obstacles .
  . presence of handrail along stairs if toilet is on another floor
  . position and functioning of door handle, faucets and flushing system
  . clear indication of men's room and ladies' room . sufficient toilet paper . position and functioning of the hand-drying machine or paper towel dispenser

√ see that visits to the toilet are made in time during car,train or air journeys

√ accompany the patient back from the toilet

**Total
take-over**

√ clearly indicate toilet door

√ fit toilet door with lock which opens from outside

√ if necessary raise toilet and fit handles in connection with restricted mobility

√ keep toilet clean

√ know about and take account of patient's previous toilet habits and continue them as far as possible

√ in the event of frequent urination at night, let the patient when sitting during the day put his feet up on a stool 8 inches (20 cm) high

√ check whether there is sufficient intake of fluids and if necessary keep note of the patient's balance of fluids

√ see that patient does not take medicines on his own initiative or try to remove feces himself with his hands

√ look out for symptoms accompanying rise in patient's temperature (above 99° F or 37° C); in these patients this can rapidly lead to greatly increased confusion, restlessness or apathy

√ consult doctor if patient complains about or there are symptoms which indicate difficulties with urinating or passing motions

Attitude

√ take (vague) complaints, signals and gestures seriously

√ be unobtrusively present and offer help if necessary

√ respect the patient's wish to go to the toilet alone and without interference (do not act simply on your own discretion; the patient's feeling of shame is still intact in stage I!)

√ realize that reproaches or annoyance about the patient dirtying himself or being careless when going to the toilet can awaken feelings of shame, depression, irritation or agression

CHAPTER 3

STAGE II

INTERVENTION

In this stage of Alzheimer's disease the mental functions have become so seriously impaired that the patient can no longer manage on his own. He needs practical help with the necessary daily routine activities at home. He functions at the comparable level of a five to seven year old child. Encouragement alone is no longer sufficient. It is now obvious even to an outsider that he has dementia. His intellectual abilities now fail him to such an extent that it interferes with maintaining himself as an independent person in the community. In terms of decline in functions of self care, this stage is characterized by the inability to choose proper clothing to wear in the way he used to. Factors such as lack of initiative and self neglect play a role. The patient lacks the ability to survey possible alternatives, to discriminate between alternatives, and to appraise the actual situation on which his choice must be based. If he makes a choice at all, the choice is impulsive and inopportune. The behavioral disturbances, which accompany the disrupted mental faculties, now also have a detrimental influence on the patient's functioning and call not only for insight but also for a great deal of tact on the part of the caregiver. While the patient may function at a level comparable to that of a six year old, he does not see the world through the eyes of a healthy, inexperienced child. He is a disabled adult who feels his control over his world slipping.

The patient himself can no longer follow the regularly recurring succession of events in his immediate surroundings. He often no longer knows the day of the week, the month or even whether it is summer or winter. It is only when he is outside that he sees snow and feels that it is cold, or he sees that there are leaves on the trees and he feels that it is warm. Sometimes he forgets where he lives. He then not only forgets the name of the street, but occasionally he does not even recognize his own house when he walks by. His own house can appear strange and unfamiliar to him. Sometimes he walks through a familiar street, but comes from a different direction than usual, and then fails to recognize it. He can no longer manage on his own outside the home and can easily get lost.

Fear of his surroundings

Visual perception itself may become disturbed, with the result that the environment can sometimes seem distorted, unfamiliar and confusing to the patient. For instance, he may sometimes have difficulty in seeing things in depth, in seeing the peripheral, which is outside his direct field of vision, or in gauging distance. The capacity to amalgamate in the mind all the details perceived by the senses into an entity, an overall picture in which everything is orderly and traceable in its appointed place, becomes disorganized. This can mean, for instance, that the patient is no longer really capable of linking the face of a person he knows to the recollection he has of that person who looks unfamiliar.

The memory for events in the patient's personal life also becomes disturbed. He can often no longer recall the name of the school he used to attend or the firm where he worked for many years. Nor can he any longer give a chronological account of his life and place the events of his life in the right order. The experiences from the past lose their relationship with one another and with the present. His brain can no longer effectively organize all the information from the outside world that is presented to it by the senses. Nor can his brain bring the memories and experiences of the past into proper alignment. The past no longer merges with the present. The patient is a prisoner in a maze of events, present and past, from which he does not know how to extricate himself. He literally loses the way in his head, as one patient expressed it. Thus it can happen that he is sometimes absolutely convinced that he is in the home of his – long deceased – parents, that his partner is one of his parents or a brother or sister, that he is still working just as he used to and that he must leave the house immediately so as not to be late.

A person's past endows the present with meaning and perspective. If all previous events and experiences which are dwelling in one's mind have been torn from their context, if the connection between past and present has been broken, then the basis of a person's own identity has been affected. When he tries to remember something, when he looks into himself, then he is confronted with increasing confusion and a growing void, since his memories are chaotic and partly erased. Being able to survey on one's life, one of the valuable assets of growing older, is impossible for the Alzheimer patient. When he looks round in his present environment for signs and points of recognition, he is confronted with an increasingly alien world. He becomes insecure and frightened and tries to orientate himself by clutching hold of whatever he can, especially another person. Many of his actions are an appeal for help to the other. That other person can still help him to structurize his increasingly chaotic world, even if it is only by being present in the same space. The patient is indeed more and more afraid of being alone. If he wakes up in the night and everything is silent and dark, there are even fewer points of contact which can form a lifeline for him. He is at times a very light sleeper and is easily wakened. Staying in bed alone may become unbearable. He must get up. Since he cannot estimate what time it is, he may no longer know whether it is now day or night.

Sometimes he clutches onto events which he knows will take place in an indeterminate future, such as going home again or going on a trip, and he keeps on asking his partner whether it is not time to go.

Sometimes he is frightened of ordinary situations, which seem to him confusing and threatening, such as the gathering darkness, and he then exhibits increasing restlessness. Or he is frightened of routine activities, which are necessary, but which he sometimes finds difficult, such as taking a shower. If he has always been a good swimmer, he is now sometimes frightened of water. Psychomotor slowing is clearly evident. Walking, especially when the patient is left to himself, becomes hesitant and groping and reflects his state of mind. In general he becomes more and more awkward in his movements.

Delusions

The patient is now increasingly subject to delusions. Delusions are false beliefs, not substantiated by sensory or objective evidence. As we have seen, distorted perception is not uncommon in Alzheimer's disease and can already occur early in its course. Consequently, delusions may be seen as attempts to find an explanation for upsetting experiences or events, which are caused by his failing memory and disturbed perception. Delusions also derive partly from lack of insight and from denial that there is anything the matter with him. At other moments reality penetrates once more and he sometimes asks anxiously: I'm not going mad, am I?" The most frequently occurring delusion in this second stage of the illness is the conviction that 'someone' is hiding his possessions away or stealing from him. He thinks that 'they' are stealing his personal belongings, since he no longer knows how and where to find them. 'They' often means his partner, his children or his caregivers. Or he believes that there are strangers who enter the house to rob him. The delusion "They are taking my possessions away from me, they are dispossessing me", is possibly connected with his experience that his mental faculties, his world, his independence are slipping away from him.

Another frequently occurring delusion is that the house where the patient is living is not his own home. 'Home' is where you feel safe and where everything is familiar. When, possibly as a result of disturbed perception and the disconnection of present and past, his own home looks different and strange, then he is not 'at home'. He therefore continually asks his caregiver to take him 'home'. Sometimes the patient's longing for his old familiar 'home' is so great that he leaves the house and goes looking outside for what he cannot find inside. This attempt is naturally doomed to failure. Outside, everything is just as confusing as it was inside. But simply through the act of walking and searching he has at least some feeling of being in control of the situation. If his partner or professional caregiver tries to stop him, that evokes agitation, rage and sometimes physical agression. This situation can be avoided by diverting him or giving him an arm and inviting him to 'go home' together with you, and walking a distance with him.

The delusion that his partner is an impostor can arise if the patient does not recognize his own partner (or professional caregiver) as such on account of disturbed perception and impaired memory. This is hurtful for the partner. A woman in the initial stage of the illness resolutely refused to go to the bedroom with her husband, because she was sure this 'strange' man had dishonorable intentions. Conversely, it also happens that the patient believes the partner is unfaithful. He or she can then become really jealous if the partner merely speaks to another man or woman. Delusions are firmly held beliefs. The patient tries to shield himself against the unbearable reality of losing control over his life. No logical argument will convince him to the contrary. It only makes him more suspicious. Many disturbing behaviors that occur in the patient with Alzheimer's disease are attempts to regain some control over one's life. Although the cause of the disturbed behavior can often not be eliminated, the anxiety and fear, which accompany and fuel it, can be substantially relieved.

In this second stage of the disease the patient often still has a notion that he is making things very difficult for his partner. The latter will sometimes express his frustration in words or gestures. It sometimes happens that the partner bursts into tears. This may bring the patient to make excuses and promises to be 'good' again. He feels helpless and guilty, and he may believe that his behavior is so bad that his partner wants to get rid of him and will send him away to a nursing home. Sometimes his own helplessness results in fits of crying with the complaint: "I want to die." One of the major problems in this stage of the disease is the patient's and the partner's inability to understand his confusion and fears. His power of speech itself is often disturbed and he is unable to find the right words to express himself. He can no longer control his emotions and is quick to scream and shout in any situation where he feels frustrated.

Undirected urge to move

In this second stage of Alzheimer's disease, the patient often still possesses a great deal of energy. If left to himself, he does not have the means to put it to constructive use. The result is that this energy is discharged in various purposeless activities, which often irritate the partner. The patient walks in and out of rooms, opens and shuts doors, takes things out of the cupboard and turns the house upside down.

The undirected activities betray an urge and need to move. They are often a continual appeal to the partner or professional caregiver to help him. Yet he often refuses to accept the offered help, he has absolutely no need of being confronted with his cognitive disability. What he does need is unobtrusive guidance. If he is allowed to perform the various necessary daily activities together with his caregiver in his own way, then he will indeed accept the offered help.

The caregiver is the only person who can draw up the scheme and planning of these activities. Apart from the necessary routine activities of personal and hygiene, there are also recreational activities. The latter can be a means of structurizing the patient's energy and urge to move and, moreover, they divert him from his fears and restlessness.

All outdoor activities, such as going shopping, taking the bus or train, going to the post office, eating in a restaurant, going to the doctor, going to the hairdresser, are completely impossible without the guidance of the caregiver.

Driving a car himself is now definitely too risky. Even though the patient often still knows how to drive, in intricate traffic situations he gets confused and takes the wrong decisions.

The more complicated activities in the home which call for any form of planning are now also impossible. Thus he no longer knows what to do with the mail and no longer has any understanding of financial affairs. He can no longer prepare even the simplest meal for himself without constant hints from, and guidance by the caregiver.

The patient can in most cases still perform the activities assoicated with personal hygiene, such as bathing, making his toilet and dressing, but only with the guidance and supervision of the caregiver. He can no longer find his own clothes. He cannot make a choice from a wardrobe full of clothing. Dressing in itself becomes an isolated procedure, which takes place without planning. In choosing his clothes the patient is unable to take account of the weather conditions, because he does not realize what they are. Under the supervision of the caregiver he can still make a choice, provided the possibilities are very limited. The best thing is for the caregiver to lay out the clothes beforehand and in the right order and let the patient dress himself. It does not really matter if dressing takes somewhat longer.

Washing also goes slowly and with interruptions, although the patient can still perform the separate actions – making himself wet, using soap, rinsing off and drying – in the right order. Usually he has to be encouraged to wash himself, under the supervision of the caregiver. It that is not done tactfully, he absolutely refuses to cooperate.

The details of daily personal hygiene, such as cleaning his teeth, shaving and doing his nails, are only performed if the patient is accompanied to the bathroom by the caregiver, all the requisites are put out within his reach beforehand and he is continually supervised and encouraged to go on by the caregiver.

Recreational pursuits are of great importance. These activities are not only aimed at keeping the patient busy, but are also intended to structurize his time and if possible maintain his functionality. In this respect each patient has his own individual possibilities and preferences. He cannot however plan or initiate these activities by himself.

Stage II, the 'guidance' or 'intervention' stage, lasts about eighteen months from the time the patient needs help with chosing, looking out and organizing his clothes to the time that the caregiver also has partially to take over dressing and undressing from the patient.

The disintegration of the mental faculties – memory, orientation, concentration, initiative and functionality – takes place according to a fairly predictable pattern. The occurrence of behavioral disturbances in the patient is less predictable. It depends on factors other than loss of cognition alone. The character and predisposition of the patient, his personal life experiences, the nature of his lifelong relationship with his partner, the ability of the caregiver to cope with the situation, all have their bearing on it.

What the patient can do himself	√ place his signature and write his name on request √ distinguish coins and bills and often name them, but without knowing the actual value √ count with comprehension from 1 to 20 and do addition and subtraction sums within this series √ distinguish between less, as much and more √ write down a named number up to 20 in figures √ at the end of stage II a number does not connote a specific amount any more to the patient; it loses its meaning as a symbol of a value
Remind and encourage patient to	√ sort money into rows or piles and then put the different coins into different glass jars √ put money in can with a slot
Intervene prevent	√ signing of official documents, checks, statements by the patient (he does not know what he is signing)
Partial take-over	√ give him money to put into a collecting-box or to pay in a shop √ let him sort different coins into glass jars √ let him add up the amount of each sort of coin
Total take-over	√ provide eight glass jars; four with a wide opening and four with a slot to put money in √ put out a number of different coins √ see that he always has some money on him to spend as he wishes
Attitude	√ respect the fact that ones own money remains important as far as it represents independence, personal possession and security. The notion of economic value ceases to exist for the patient, who now can no longer control his financial affairs. The urge to hold on to one's money however is very deep-seated. The patient feels his possessions gradually being taken away from him and resists every act of dispossession. Perhaps he will retain more faith in the management of his money by the caregiver, if he is allowed to handle limited sums of money by himself.

What the patient can do himself	√ sometimes still able to answer the door bell √ open and shut the front door and lock it √ pass things round without missing anyone out √ carry out simple tasks (see **stage II the kitchen**)
Remind and encourage patient to if necessary explain step by step	carry out the above-mentioned acts by: √ pointing to something and say in a friendly tone: "Open – the front door" "Shut – the door; lock – the door" "Pick up that dish – hand on to everyone"
Intervene observe for, if necessary prevent	√ inability of the patient to react to a request; he can usually carry it out step by step if guided as follows: first direct his attention to the object: "Do you see that glass? Could you give it to me?" Then: "Will you take it to the kitchen?"
Partial take-over	√ check whether the front door is locked
Total take-over	√ general supervision of all tasks given √ serving of all alcoholic beverages
Attitude	√ keep the patient involved in the conversation; for instance, say repeatedly: "That's right, isn't it, John?" Act as intermediary between him and the visitor; help the patient when he is trying to say something, so as to keep the conversation going

What the patient can do himself	√ pick flowers √ dig holes √ rake up leaves and twigs √ use his hands to fill and empty the wheelbarrow √ push the wheelbarrow and keep it on an even keel √ in previously prepared ground, put bulbs into holes and cover them with earth √ use a watering can
Remind and encourage patient to if necessary explain step by step	√ carry out simple acts which he can do himself by pointing to things and saying in a friendly manner: "You see those flowers – will you pick them..." "Pick up that spade – dig out some earth..." "Take that broom – sweep..." "Pick that up – put it in ..." "Pick up – lift up with both hands – push ..." "Pick up that bulb – put it in the hole – cover it over ..." "Pick that up – water those things – stop ..." √ putting on shoes or rubber boots
Intervene observe for and prevent	√ walking away and getting lost; (he may sometimes fail to recognize his own garden) √ unsafe use of garden tools √ the wheelbarrow capsizing
Partial take-over	√ take the flowers which he has picked √ indicate size and depth of hole to be dug √ turn the wheelbarrow in the right direction √ fill the watering can – indicate where to water
Total take-over	√ see to the maintenance of the garden & garden tools √ store all garden implements out of his reach √ put out sturdy shoes or rubber boots √ get rid of poisonous or otherwise harmful plants
Attitude	√ show appreciation of his achievements √ continue to emphasize that it is 'his' garden

What the patient can do himself	√ take part in simple joint activities in a small group (not more than six people) under someones direction
	√ work with visible quantities
	√ count from 1 to 20 and associate these numbers with a certain quantity
	√ distinguish relative quantities and locations: more, less and as much; forwards and backwards; left and right; above and below; next to, on and under; fast and slow
	√ take part in games and other communal activities which call for a regularly changing order of participation
	√ take his turn in throwing two dice and naming the value of his throw and then moving his counter/chip
	√ play his musical instrument
Remind and encourage patient to if necessary explain step by step	√ go on with recreational activities
	√ participate in group activities inside and outside the family, in the house and out of the house
	√ keep his attention on the game
	√ take action when it is his turn; wait for his turn
Intervene observe for and if necessary prevent	√ difficulty in adjusting himself to the game, to the material, the space and the movements required for the game
	√ restlessness and increased urge to move resulting from frustration, disagreement and argument between the patient and his fellow players
Partial take-over	√ see that the conversation is carried on in simple sentences and at a normal pitch; there are often attempts by means of speaking more quickly or in a more lively way to obtain more reactions from the patient, which can lead to agitation; stimulate the conversation and keep it going; give the patient his glasses and put on his hearing aid
	√ provide him with the musical instrument of his choice and see to it that it is in proper condition

Total take-over

√ choose recreational activities which are suited to the capacities of the patient

√ in general less suitable games are those in which: instructions have to be read and followed all the time; constant concentration is called for; there is great emphasis on competition; a variety of details have to be remembered all the time

√ make up groups of not more than six players per leader

√ see to:
  . safe activities and a safe environment
  . restful and attractive surroundings
  . interaction amongst the players and between leader and players
  . sufficient attention for each individual patient
  . good quality material suited to adults
  . variety in recreational activities

Attitude

√ realize that playing a game is something which everyone enjoys and needs to do, both young and old. Within the game the patient can safely devote himself to the activity – there is no compulsion or necessity. He is allowed and able to lose himself in a game. The relaxed atmosphere of the game and the fact of doing something together with other people can strengthen his self-assurance

√ at least one day a week undertake a physical exercise activity with the patient outside the house

√ choose the right moment to ask the patient to make music. Never force a recreational activity on him. In order to be able to concentrate on something, he needs all the attention and consideration of those around him

What the patient can do himself	√ form the separate elements of a compound word into one word √ read compound words √ connect a word he has read with an illustration relating to that word √ connect the first part of a compound word with the corresponding illustration and the second part of the compound word with or without the corresponding illustration
Remind and encourage patient to if necessary explain step by step	√ choose and join up the corresponding part of the word
Intervene observe for if necessary prevent	√ discouragement and frustration resulting from inability to find the right combination
Partial take-over	√ choose and hand over the first part of a compound word √ let the patient choose from not more than four parts of words for the second part of the word to be formed √ begin with the word blocks, without illustration √ let him do the exercise whereby both blocks which constitute the compound word have the word plus the corresponding illustration; then only put out the first part with corresponding illustration and let him choose the second part without the illustration √ put out four blocks with illustrations and give him one of the four corresponding pictures and ask: "Where does this belong?" if necessary point to the picture in his hand √ if necessary demonstrate to show him what the intention is

Total take-over

√ design material for broken word connections:
1. collect compound words, each part of which is illustrated separately, such as: wrist-watch, note-paper, bath-robe, swim-suit, tooth-paste, bird-cage, pen-knife, shoe-horn, snow-ball, pig-pen, door-mat, fire-place, fisher-man, flower-pot, motor-bike
2. make two sorts of block, each 2 x 5 cm (or 1x2 inches); one sort with part of a compound word without the illustration belonging to it, and one sort with part of a compound word with the corresponding picture, measuring 5 x 8 cm (or 2x3 inches) design clear, colored illustrations such as:
egg – egg cup, baby – baby carriage, flower – vase, bird – nest, snail – snail's shell, apple – tree, fork – knife + spoon, skirt – blouse, teeth – brush, spider – web, bath – towel, mouse – mousetrap, butterfly – net, football – boot/helmet .
comb – head of hair, bath/shower – naked figure/soap

√ stick the pictures onto a hard base of at least 10 x 10 cm (or 4 x 4 inches)

What the patient can do himself	√ play cards; provided he is an experienced card player, he can join in simple, familiar games
	√ deal, shuffle, cut, or take from a pack of cards
	√ do a jigsaw puzzle consisting of approximately twenty reasonably large pieces in a frame, by trial and error
Encourage patient to if necessary explain step by step	√ continue with playing games and doing puzzles
	√ do puzzles: take the lid off the box; look at the picture: name the objects in the picture; take the puzzle apart; lay the pieces out at randomwith the colored side up; put the puzzle together within the frame
Intervene observe for	√ discouragement and frustration because of inaptitude
Partial take-over	√ see that there is a suitable cards partner who knows the patient's condition and is accepted by the patient
Total take-over	√ devise suitable recreational activities; choose an activity which most closely matches his preference and special skills
	√ determine the right moment for an activity, bearing in mind his mood, energy and inclination
	√ provide a quiet environment; no disturbing sound from TV or radio
	√ use materials known to the patient – give a short and clear explanation and a demonstration
	√ determine the optimal duration of activity – not too long, not too short
Attitude	√ realize that it is not enough only to suggest an activity to the patient; frequently he cannot clearly picture it, which is often the reason for lack of activity in the patient
	√ he cannot occupy himself without help; during the game he must be constantly encouraged. But he must also retain his freedom to act as he wishes as far aspossible
	√ realize that he will make mistakes. If he is often reminded of mistakes, he feels that people are criticizing him, which can result in anger, tears and discouragement

What the patient can do himself

√ make music and sing:
  . look at and listen to a performance of music and singing
  . make music on his own instrument
  . sing or join in singing songs he has known from the past
  . rhythmically move his body to the beat of the music
  . join in singing in church

Encourage to
if necessary explain

√ join in singing
√ join in clapping
√ sway to the rhythm while seated; arm in arm with partner

Intervene
observe for

√ signs of pleasure or anxiety

Partial take-over

√ hand him his instrument or take him to it

Total take-over

√ find out what sort of music appeals to him at particular times. Music with a pronounced rhythm stimulates movement, quiet listening music has a calming influence. Playing or singing music familiar to the patient gives him a feeling of security. Past experiences can be recalled through music and movements
√ in making music adjust type of music, tempo and volume to the patient and not to the caregiver
√ see that his instrument is in working order
√ accompany the patient to musical performances, such as concerts, musicals, opera

Attitude

√ bear in mind and see to it that the patient does not get music or singing 'lessons'. He must be entirely free in his reaction to and participation in music and singing
√ empathize with and appreciate the way in which he experiences and makes music

What the patient can do himself

√ cut out; cut away the superfluous paper round a simple, reasonably large figure with scissors
√ paste figures cut from paper onto a sheet of drawing paper and collect the sheets in a file or portfolio
√ leaf through the portfolio recognizing what he sees as his own creation

Remind and encourage patient to
if necessary explain

√ choose the paper figures; cut them out; put on glue; stick them on
√ explain a collage he has made himself
√ regularly look through his portfolio

Intervene
observe for and if necessary prevent

√ hurting himself: use paper-cutting scissors
√ frustration and irritation when something goes wrong
√ if he cannot manage the cutting out, take it over from him

Partial take-over

√ stimulate patient to make collages:
  . as a means of self expression
  . as free expression
  . as a paricular assignment
√ provide all the necessary material
√ explain the activity
√ use the collages he has made as explanatory material:
  . in order to illustrate beforehand an action which he has to perform, for instance, discussing the pictures of the bathroom with him before bathing
  . as an aid to the expression of his feelings or thoughts: join with the patient in composing a collage

**Total
take-over**

√ take the initiative for the patient of being creatively occupied

√ provide ideas for a scrapbook with pictures, and help compile
  . find out if he has special interests, e.g. birds, fish, pets, insects, plants, flowers, 'planes, cars, trains, stamps, interiors such as bed- sitting rooms, bathrooms, kitchens
  . collect the necessary material from magazines, leaflets, photos. An image must measure at least 5 x 8 cm (2,5 x 3,5 inches) and be colorful.

√ provide a loose-leaf file for the collages so that additions can easily be inserted

√ purchase sheets of stiff paper 50 x 30 cm (20 x 12 inches)

√ keep up the collection of pictures

√ show his work to family and friends

Attitude

√ Realize that making collages can be a means of expressing experiences which can no longer be put into words; isolated images are formed into an entity. Collages can provide the caregiver with insight into the way the patient thinks and help document his changing world

What the patient can do himself	√ use a pencil, pen, paintbrush √ draw and sometimes copy highly simplified figures with pen, pencil, felt tip pen √ color: work with a limited number of colors: red, yellow, blue, green, black √ use brushes of different thicknesses: dip into the paint, wipe off, brush onto paper and rinse in the fluid
Encourage patient to if necessary explain step by step	√ draw spontaneously √ draw particular figures: house, tree, person √ put his name and the date on the drawing or painting
Partial take-over	√ take the initiative for the activity √ provide the proper materials √ fix the sheet of drawing paper on a drawing board (shifting paper is discouraging) √ discuss objects of interest to the patient with him and let him discuss his work √ give him his own folder in which to keep his work
Total take-over	√ provide the opportunity for him to work in his own way, according to his mental capacities and preferences and at his own pace √ select materials: non-toxic paint and pencils; thicker pencils/crayons with hard tip √ give small quantities of paint; if there is a lot of paint, he puts the brush right in, so that the paint drips off the handle
Attitude	√ choose actions and activities which do not overtax or underestimate the patient's capabilities and take care not to correct his 'faults'. This incites frustration, agitation and sometimes anger √ quietly allow him to find his own way

**What the
patient can
do himself**

√ work with modeling clay or dough, i.e.:
   knead, press, slap, bore holes, cut pieces off,
   roll and turn

Encourage to
if necessary
explain
step by step

√ occupy himself with clay or dough
√ knead well
√ use a pallet to cut pieces off

**Partial
take-over**

√ knead the clay once before use; give the patient
   a preferably shapeless lump of clay, so that he can make
   whatever he wants to
√ suggest a shape if the patient himself cannot think of
   anything

**Total
take-over**

√ choice of materials; clay should not be too
   hard and be sufficiently pliable
√ if the patient or caregiver dislikes working with clay,
   then dough is to be recommended; it does not stain. To
   make the dough mix 500 gram flour (17,5 ounces) and
   100 gram (3,5 ounces) salt, add water until there is a
   pliable substance which is not sticky (for two people).
   Keep the dough in a tightly closed pot.

Attitude

√ participate in the modeling, but let the patient go
   ahead without interference. The emphasis is on
   modeling together; never give him the impression that
   the aim of the activity is to 'keep him quiet'
√ realize that clay or dough invite manipulation with the
   hands. This stimulates the sense of touch and exercises
   the fine finger movements as well as the coordinated
   use of both hands

What the patient can do himself

√ using the loose pieces, put together and take apart construction components by means of:
  . screwing; wind the nut spirally round the thread
  . pushing; get pieces to engage by pressing
  . fitting a tongue into a groove, thus connecting two pieces up into one, e.g. a hoop
  . allowing two pieces to engage one another by means of a coupling
√ pick up metal parts with a magnet

Encourage to Intervene observe for and if necessary prevent

√ work with construction boxes
√ frustration: if a technique cannot be mastered, it can be very disheartening
√ lack of patience and irritation when something does not work
√ quickly giving up an activity

Partial take-over

√ offer a variety of construction components and observe which actions cause him the most difficulty
√ demonstrate the various techniques of putting together the two parts, if necessary

Total take-over

√ buy durable and robust construction material; plastic material from a toyshop is often rejected by the patient
√ building with plastic material is more successful and enjoyable if done with a grandchild

What the patient can do himself	√ go for a walk along walking trails in the woods and hills, and along the beach √ shuffle through the leaves in the fall √ sit at the water's edge and feed the ducks √ enjoy the view √ name some of the plants, flowers or animals √ pick flowers and collect shells √ dabble on the beach √ push a grandchild in a carriage √ cycle along paved bicycle paths
Remind and encourage the patient if necessary explain	√ wear clothes suitable for the activity; for instance, put on a loosely fitting sweatsuit √ undertake activities such as picking flowers, feeding ducks
Intervene observe for and if necessary prevent	√ stumbling √ slippery surface √ picking poisonous plants or berries √ straying or getting lost
Partial take-over	√ point out flora and fauna and ask the patient to name them or tell something about them √ provide bucket or basket for collecting shells, nuts, fruit etc. Collected items can be utilized at home to: . relive the walk . sort out into kind, size or put into rows or piles √ avoid overexposure to the sun
Total take-over	√ do not tell him about an outdoor activity long beforehand; this avoids continual questioning: "When are we going?" √ regularly going out for walks together at set times in the evening before going to bed can have a favorable influence on restlessness and increased urge to be active in the evening and can also be beneficial in promoting sleep

What the patient can do himself

√ provided that he is an experienced swimmer:
  . float
  . breaststroke
  . backstroke
√ for swimmers who have previously participated in aquatic gymnastics in shallow water:
  . in upright position imitate exercises with arms and legs performed by an instructor
  . walk with or throw a large ball
√ undress himself in the locker room
√ put on his swimsuit in the locker room
√ take a shower
√ dress himself in the locker room

Remind and encourage patient to
if necessary
explain
step by step

√ go to the toilet before swimming
√ change in the locker room
√ put on bathing shoes (no mules) which cover the heel and with nonslip soles
√ put on bath wrap or wrap bath towel around his body
√ shower before and after aquatic activitiy
√ go with him into the water (do not force him)
√ after swimming, take off swimsuit, get dry and get dressed in the locker room

Intervene
observe for
and if neces-
sary prevent

√ spatial orientation in the locker room and swimming pool
√ sudden fear and confusion resulting from insecurity
√ losing his footing on slippery floor
√ lack of breath during swimming or exercises (urge him to breathe deeply and regularly)
√ rapid reduction of the body temperature continued shivering
√ bumping his head against the edge of the pool
√ evidence or complaints of:
  . fatigue
  . tightness of the chest
  . dizziness
  . reacting slower than normal
√ suddenly jumping or diving into the water
√ not being able to find his clothes any more

Partial take-over	√ hang up his clothes or give them to the attendant
	√ go under the shower with him
	√ after showering give him his hand towel and clothes

Total take-over

√ see that aquatic gymnastics and swimming take place exclusively in water at a temperature of about 30 degrees. This relaxes muscles and joints, promotes mental relaxation, keeps the body temperature stable and promotes better blood flow of the muscles

√ do not let him take part in aquatic activities in the event of conditions such as:
. fear and panic
. a cold or allergic reactions
. serious skin disorders
. incontinence
. high blood pressure
. perforated eardrum

√ let the bath superintendent know about the patient's condition: continuous supervision is called for

√ if necessary ask swimming pool staff for help with changing

√ put swimming requisites out ready

√ accompany patient to swimming pool

√ buy admission ticket, escort him to separate locker room and pool

√ check in with and greet swimming/gymnastics instructor

√ accompany patient to shower

√ adjust shower faucets to slightly more than lukewarm water

√ accompany patient from the broad steps into the shallow water

√ after the aquatic activity hand out bath robe or towel to prevent cooling off

Attitude

√ put the emphasis on the sportive element and the experience of pleasure, not on the patient's ability to do things perfectly. Being pleasurably active without danger, mitigates and avoids tension and fear, whereby at the same time motor skills are improved or maintained

What the patient can do himself

√ in a group of six patients, plus the leader of the dancing, join in the movements of a round dance or row dance
√ perform familiar dances with or without guidance
√ change partners during the dance if a hand is invitingly extended
√ on command:
  . go and stand in the square or row
  . stand still
  . begin with the right foot
  . take the partner(s) by the right/left hand
  . put his hands to his waist
  . put hands on each other's shoulders
  . do side step-close-side step
  . take one to three steps forward and the same number of steps backward
  . move freely through the room to the beat of the music
√ imitate movements:
  . stand on one leg and make side step-close-side step movements
  . raise his leg and put his foot forward or to the side
  . arm in arm together with his partner, dance round in a small circle
  . join in walking round, hand in hand, in a circle
  . join in walking in a line with hands on each other's shoulders

Remind and encourage

√ go to the toilet before the activity
√ join in, moving to the music

Intervene observe for and if necessary prevent

√ lack of concentration and willingness on the part of the patient to participate (time of day and mood of patient may be of influence)
√ see to:
  . patient wearing his glasses and his hearing aid when necessary
  . patient wearing well-fitting shoes with nonslip soles and heels and loosely fitting clothes
  . stamina, respiration and equilibrium while dancing

Partial take-over

√ take the initiative to move to the music
√ allow patient to dance spontaneously
√ avoid frequently correcting the patient in words or gestures. This may engender confusion and can cause falls or agitation
√ indicate rhythm by means of counting
√ while dancing in couples (patient and healthy partner) unobtrusively correct the rhythm of his arm and feet movements
√ while dancing maintain continual contact with him; a large hall can have a confusing effect while dancing

Total take-over

√ create a secure environment:
. see that the room is well-lit and has a not too slippery floor
. comfortable room temperature
. enough chairs
. enough non-patient dance partners
. avoid dances with which the patient is not familiar or does not like
. arrange for music with not too fast a rhythm, with which the patient is familiar
. avoid too loud music which irritates the patient
. arrange groups of not more than six patients per leader

Attitude

√ experience pleasure together in moving to music
√ realize that it is most important *that* the patient moves to music, not *how* he moves
√ accept the situation if the patient stops dancing and just goes on walking. Allow him to stop when he wants to
√ patting him on the back or caressing him has a stimulating and encouraging effect

What the patient can do himself

√ throw and fling various sorts of balls and quoits (flat plastic rings)

√ catch a ball at a short distance and throw it back

√ sitting opposite a fellow player, a ball or other suitable object can be:
  . thrown underhand
  . passed over underhand, overhand or crosswise

√ sitting opposite a fellow player a ball or other suitable object can simultaneously with him be:
  . thrown from one hand to the other
  . put from one hand into the other under his raised upper leg or round the bottom of his back

Encourage patient to

√ continue to throw and catch

Intervene observe for and prevent

√ loss of balance when trying to catch the ball or ring

√ fatigue or loss of interest and concentration; these are a reason to end the game

Partial take-over

√ let the patient choose the object to be thrown, i.e., ball or ring

Total take-over

√ obtain suitable articles to throw:
  . colored balls of various sizes
  . make cloth bags of 10 x 20 cm (4 x 8 inches), filled with brown beans or haricot beans, to throw to and fro

√ casually increase and decrease the distance to be thrown while both players are seated

Attitude

√ show genuine interest in the patient's activities Questions such as:"Do you like it?" "Is it going well?" encourage him because the patient feels his partner also enjoys the game. The ball game is a form of non-threatening, quasi-competitive, unconstrained contact between the patient and his partner. It promotes concentration and stimulates coordinated movements

What the patient can do himself	√ play with a coil of rope, standing or sitting: . take hold of it . keep hold of it . swing it to and fro, in front of and to the side of the body . let it slide through his hands . move it from one hand to the other . put it over his head like a chain and take it off again . tug-of-war or swinging rope to and fro with a fellow player
Encourage patient to	√ swing it to and fro, pull harder or less hard √ take it in turns to pull hard while both hold onto the rope √ take the fellow player in tow √ be taken in tow by the fellow player
Intervene observe for and prevent	√ the pace being raised too quickly √ wobbling on account of fatigue or loss of balance √ roughening of the game
Partial take-over	√ if possible, accompany the exercises with singing or music √ take it in turn to determine the rhythm of the movements or let the patient determine it
Total take-over	√ buy a rope of cotton fiber 180 cm (72 inches)long and without bulges. The ends are plaited together so that it forms a circle √ do the exercises together in a relaxed and playful manner
Attitude	√ realize that playing with a rope promotes the locomotor adjustment to the fellow player

What the patient can do himself	√ play with a hoop, standing or sitting: . take hold of it . keep hold of it . put it vertically on the ground in front of him . hold it with two hands in front of him horizontally . in the vertical position push it through his hands or let it slide through . let his hands slide as far as a certain color segment . put from one hand to the other on a certain color . move it to and fro with two hands . move it above his head . put the hoop flat on the ground and step in and out of it . trail a large hoop over the ground behind him
Encourage patient to	√ perform the various movements with the hoop √ look at and imitate movements of his fellow player
Intervene observe for and prevent	√ threatening loss of equilibrium (in that case do the exercises sitting down) √ shortage of breath during exertion (urge him to breathe deeply and slowly)
Partial take-over	√ hand over the hoop
Total take-over	√ see that there are hoops: . a hoop 70 cm (28 inches) in diameter, consisting of four equally large colored segments in red, green, blue and yellow . a hoop 100 cm (40 inches) in diameter, which he can trail behind him over the ground
Attitude	√ realize that: . playing with the hoop promotes coordinated movements . the time of day and the patient's mood influence his exertions and concentration

What the patient can do himself

√ play with a club made of lightweight material, as used for gymnastic exercises:
  . take hold of it
  . keep hold of it
  . walking or sitting swing the club from the wrist and shoulder
  . move the club from one hand to another
  . swing to and fro in front of and sideways from the body
  . raise the club with two hands round the thick part
  . in pairs (patient and caregiver) sitting opposite each other tap one another's club

Encourage patient to

√ pick up the club by the neck
√ walk, stand still or sit down with the club in the hand
√ imitate the movements of the fellow player

observe for and prevent

√ fatigue, irritation or agitation are reason to end the game
√ hitting with the club

Partial take-over

√ see that club is taken hold of by the neck during the exercise
√ go along with the movements of the patient

Total take-over

√ obtain clubs made of lightweight material
√ see that there is a safe environment to minimize the chance of falls
√ avert patient walking backwards – this can lead to falls
√ make sure the patient can handle the club and is not in an agressive mood

Attitude

√ as for ball, rope and hoop games
√ see that the patient does not learn any wrong movements and is never forced into action which he does not want

What the patient can do himself	√ perform most simple single actions on request √ turn a faucet on and off √ wash his hands √ name household activities and objects √ put tableware on the table and clear a laid table; one object at a time in both hands √ make the bed – strip the bed √ water the flowers √ wash down or dust drainboard or furniture √ hold a trash bag or door open √ hang up and fold up washing √ empty a cupboard shelf; (but not putting things back again) √ rinse washing – wring out dishcloth
Remind and encourage patient to if necessary explain step by step	√ start and carry out an activity; always relate the activity requested from the patient to a concrete situation; give simple instructions in a friendly tone, i.e.: . "put on the table – two plates – two cups and saucers" . "make the bed – straighten the sheet" . "give that plant water – that one too" . "sweep the crumbs – from this table" . "hold the door open – hold this trash bag open" . "hang this coat on that hook" – "hang this washing on the line" . "take those things out of that cupboard" . "rinse this washing"
Intervene observe for and if necessary prevent	√ requesting complicated actions from the patient. The goal of an action escapes him, but if he is given an object, accompanied by a simple instructions, he can often use it correctly in a concrete situation √ activities requiring the use of tools: the patient can no longer use tools effectively. Usually he can still connect two every day objects through *one* action, e.g.: watering a plant with a watering can; washing his hands with soap and drying them with a hand towel

Intervene   √ the occurrence of adverse reactions to sounds, such as
the doorbell, telephone, whistling kettle, car horn,
running water and the mewing of the cat. At the end of
stage II these sounds are simply heard, but no longer
linked to the source. This leads either to ignoring the
sound or to panic reactions. Both can be dangerous

Partial   √ at the beginning of an activity, name and explain
take-over   the action in simple terms and at the same time show
or give the patient the required object
√ put the objects, needed for the action, within his reach
or hand them to him, for instance:
. a basket of wet washing to be hung up and clothes
pins
. one sort of cloth to be folded up
. a duster or dishtowel
. a bowl filled with water, in which to rinse something

Total   √ let him work without disturbing noises, such as
take-over   blaring sounds from radio and TV
√ put the emphasis on doing together complicated
activities, such as changing a bed
√ from time to time play a subservient role. Ask the
patient: "What would you like me to clean today?" A
little later say: "Can you tell me how to do it?" this
reinforces his self esteem

Attitude   √ notice that fear and desperation may occur if he has to
carry out too complicated a task
√ watch out that:
. he does not get the feeling that the control over the
household is being totally taken over by someone
else. This can lead to his not looking after anything
any more, or in resistance
. the caregiver should avoid demonstratively redoing
the work the patient has just done. This may cause
confusion, discouragement and negativism in the
patient. The necessary corrections can be made later
by the caregiver

What the patient can do himself	*up to about halfway stage II:* √ go to a familiar local shop without having to cross the street √ hand over a short shopping list and money to the shopkeeper or sales clerk √ wait for his turn provided he is kept occupied √ put the purchases in a shopping bag or shopping cart and take them home √ take money out of and put into his purse
Remind and encourage patient to	√ hand over the shopping list to the shopkeeper √ come home again after the shopping
Intervene observe for and if necessary prevent	√ shopping without a list √ incorrect payment (the patient does not know if he should have change or not) √ distraction and going astray (the patient is easily distracted by unexpected events which attract his attention) √ forgetting the object of the exercise, becoming panic stricken and subsequently unable to find the way home √ on impulse do other things such as walking away, getting onto a bus, streetcar or subway train
Partial take-over	√ before shopping, give him: . a shopping list . exact money . a carrying bag or shopping cart
Total take-over	√ if necessary keep an eye on him from a distance √ let the shopkeeper know that the patient needs help with shopping and paying for the purchases
Attitude	√ take account of the patient's feeling of self- esteem. If he walks in the wrong direction, quietly walk towards him and give him an encouraging pat on the back, saying: "I'm going shopping too. Are you coming shopping with me?" or "Let's have a cup of coffee."

What the patient can do himself

√ recognize and partially name familiar kitchen equipment and utensils

√ on request gather up to ten items, e.g., apples, eggs etc.

√ put an item away in an indicated place

√ take an item from the person who hands it to him

√ hand somebody an item on request

√ on request get familiar, clearly displayed products out of the refrigerator

√ pour liquid from a container into a wide glass or bowl

√ dish up from a pan onto a plate

√ shake the contents out of a packet or bag

√ pour or scoop a certain amount of a substance into or out of a receptacle

√ wash and reasonably wipe non-fragile objects

√ top and tail and/or shell green beans, broad beans, peas etc.

√ perform most simple, familiar actions such as: wiping up; pouring out; kneading; scooping out; picking up with a fork; stirring; peeling; cutting into pieces; squeezing; throwing away

Remind and encourage patient to
if necessary explain step by step

√ begin an activity

√ go on with the activity:

√ caregiver indicates an object and says in a friendly way

. take this cloth – wipe up

. take that glass – pour out (if necessary stop)

. press – knead – the dough well

. take this spoon – scoop everything out

. take this spoon – stir the pan – gently

. take this meat – roll it in your hands (portions of ground meat)

. take that (e.g. lemon) – squeeze – into a glass

. take that (e.g. garbage) – throw into garbage can

Intervene
observe for
and if neces-
sary prevent

√ inability to finish an activity; observe whether
   the patient can connect two objects, required for
   a particular action, with one another,
   can subsequently perform the action requested, and can
   complete the activity in its totality
√ understand the purpose of a particular action
√ frustration when he is unable to perform an activity
   satisfactorily

**Partial
take-over**

√ give the patient measured and weighed quantities
   of necessary requisites
√ fill a pan half-full of water and put this on a nonslip
   mat within his reach
√ use of the hot water faucet
√ use of all kitchen appliances, i.e., microwave oven,
   stove, dishwasher, washer, food processor, coffee mill.
   The patient can no longer operate these appliances
   safely on his own

**Total
take-over**

√ let him frequently perform familiar routine actions
√ the final supervision of all activities
√ see that the kitchen is arranged in an orderly way with
   a view to the actions and activities to be carried out by
   the patient
√ put matches and potentially harmful substances out of
   reach
√ operate the stove
√ remove tainted food
√ see that there is a fairly sharp knife with a broad handle
   and a rounded edge
√ immediately dry off a wet floor to prevent sliding
√ clean the garbage can
√ wipe knives, forks and glassware

Attitude

√ take into account that the patient can no longer do things requiring a change of strategy. He can only do things in the old, well-tried way. If difficulties arise during the action, he cannot find solutions

√ accept the fact that he does everything slowly and stops if he does not wish to go on or does not know how to

√ show respect for the way in which he carries out an activity: he does things in his own way

√ take into account that he breaks off the activity if people do not continually involve him in it

√ say appreciative things to the patient, such as: "You're a good cook, teach me to cook like that." "May I help you?"

What the patient can do himself

√ recognize, name and point to in himself and in someone else certain external parts of the body:
. head, ears, eyes, nose, lips, tongue and hair
. stomach, back and buttocks
. arm, hand, fingers (only thumb and little finger)
. leg, knee, foot, toes

√ indicate the functions of the body parts:
. nose – smell
. ears – hear
. eyes- see
. mouth – eat, talk, kiss
. hand – grasp, smack, fondle
. foot and leg – walk, kick

√ distinguish between:
. left and right
. above and below
. in front and behind

Encourage patient to

√ name parts of his body: while helping with bathing and dressing, touch one part of the body and name it simultaneously e.g. the left foot. Directly afterwards ask: "Show me your left foot' or "What am I stroking?"

Intervene

√ use a doll or image of a human body for a body scheme exercise if the patient finds the doll too childish, do not use it)

**Partial
take-over**

√ body scheme exercises: first point to parts of
body and then let patient name them. Or point to
them, name them and let the patient repeat them.
Subsequently ask patient to point to these parts of the
body on the partner

√ exercises with aid of a body scheme puzzle (see chapter
2, **Body scheme**):

. at the front and back of the figure, first point to the
parts and then let patient name them. Or point and
name and let him repeat what has been named

. have the patient take the parts out one by one:
caregiver says: "Give me a leg". (Since the patient can
no longer understand the reversal of right and left in
the mirror image, do not ask for right and left parts
from the puzzle)

. help him to put the parts together, without his having
to name them

**Total
take-over**

√ see chapter 2, **Body scheme**, for how to construct
a body figure puzzle

√ before and during bathing and dressing are suitable
times at which to casually perform body scheme
exercises as mentioned above

√ with regard to recognition, naming and indication of
parts of the body, it is sometimes worthwhile using a
baby-sized doll alongside or instead of the puzzle

Attitude

√ take into account that at the end of stage II conscious
orientation disappears. Practicing the body concept can
help the patient in the performance of the habitual
actions of bathing and dressing himself

What the patient can do himself

√ orientate himself in his own bathroom
√ use familiar toilet requisites within his reach
√ turn the faucet on and off
√ unscrew a bottle
√ step into the bath tub, sit down in the bath tub and wash the parts of the body above the surface of the water and subsequently the lower part of the body
√ stand under the shower, draw the shower curtain, soap his upper body as far as the private parts and rinse the soap off
√ wash himself at the washbasin with the exception of his back, legs and feet
√ dry his whole body seated
√ hang up the used bath towel

Remind and encourage patient to
if necessary explain step by step

√ go to the bathroom, take off his dressing gown, bedroom slippers and put them in the appropriate place
√ get into the bath tub and sit down
√ step into the shower, draw the shower curtain and sit on the shower chair
√ make himself thoroughly wet under the shower
√ pick up washcloth and soap, put soap on washcloth and soap himself
√ if necessary hold onto handrail
√ wash the parts of the body; name them one by one
√ step out of the bath or shower
√ dry himself with the hand towel
√ rub in the body lotion (applied by the caretaker)

Intervene
observe for and if necessary prevent

√ see stage I, Bathing and skin care, Intervene and observe for
√ patient's comprehension of the ongoing action (notice whether he can make the connection between soap-washcloth, washcloth-body and hand towel-body)
√ slipping and falling
√ soap getting in his eyes, which makes him frightened

Partial take-over

√ where necessary: hand him a soaped washcloth and make washing movements; wash his back, legs and feet; wash his neck and ears; rinse off remains of soap; help dry skin folds

√ apply lotion to a part of the body (patient can rub it in himself)

Total take-over

√ the supervision of daily care of the body. The notion of personal hygiene disappears during this stage

√ make preparations for the total activity:
. get the bathroom to the right temperature
. put out his familiar requisites within reach
. put nonslip mats on the floor in bathtub/shower
. place a chair in the bathtub or shower
. put clothes out ready
. run water into bathtub or washbasin

√ get shower water to the right temperature and let it run gently before the patient stands under it (an unexpectedly strong jet of too cold or too hot water frightens him)

√ when using a hand shower, which is preferable, first invite the patient to sit on the shower chair and then turn on the water

√ apply deodorant in the armpits

Attitude

√ see stage I Personal care & hygiene, bathing & skin care

√ choose the right moment to encourage him to shower, bathe or wash; he may no longer know the purpose of these activities

√ realize that there are various reasons for being frightened of bathing in stage II: slipping and falling; finding it difficult to move in a confined space; being alone in a closed off space

√ fear of bathing can often be obviated if the partner also goes under the shower

√ forcing the patient to bathe or shower never leads to the intended goal; it only increases his resistance

√ see that the total activity takes place in a restful atmosphere. If the patient is hurried up too much, muscular tension, fear, irritation and defensive reactions can occur

What the patient can do himself
√ perform simple unsophisticated but independent movements with each of his fingers
√ on request stretch out the left or right hand
√ name his fingers separately (thumb...etc)
√ wash and dry his hands
√ unscrew the cap of a bottle, take the lid off a box (but not always put it on)
√ squeeze cream out of a tube or take it out of a pot and rub into his hands

Remind and encourage to
√ wash his hands with soap
√ apply hand cream and rub it in

Intervene
observe for, if necessary and when possible prevent
√ dirty hands and nails; dry, brittle nails
√ sharp, protruding edges of nails
√ frayed cuticles; inflamed cuticles
√ chapped hands
√ cuts; skin rash; eczema
√ painful and swollen finger and wrist joints

Partial
√ see to it that the patient washes his hands after going to the toilet, meals and other activities

Total take-over
√ put out hand towel and soap
√ clean fingernails
√ cut, file nails; keep cuticles loose
√ daily finger exercise by massaging the back of the hand and the fingers one by one and simultaneously stretching them. Inactive fingers can be subject to malformation
√ provide skin cream to keep hands and fingers supple

Attitude
√ the hands are the principal instrument for the sense of touch, the sense which continues to function the longest. His hands become the patient's most important connection with the surrounding world in stages III and IV
√ neglect of hands and nails can lead to skin infections or gastrointestinal complaints
√ painful joints can lead to premature loss of function in the hands

What the patient can do himself

√ in seated position:
- wash and dry his feet
- put on shoes, tights, socks, panty hose
- on request show his left or right foot

√ distinguish the left and right shoe

Remind and encourage patient to

√ wash his feet in seated position in bathtub or shower cabin; use washcloth and soap; put soap on washcloth; wash feet, also between the toes; rinse feet; dry feet and toes; put on panty hose, socks and shoes in seated position

Intervene observe for and if necessary prevent

√ possible problems when bending forward (also when seated), such as: loss of equilibrium; shortness of breath; giddiness (clutching his head with his hand or holding on to something)

√ wearing comfortable shoes instead of bedroom slippers for:
- better balance
- better ability to lift up feet
- better relaxation of the calf muscle
- better protection of the feet

Partial take-over

√ help to see that feet are really dry

√ if necessary lay his footwear out for him or hand him the shoe and indicate which shoe belongs to which foot

√ tie the shoelaces when necessary

Total take-over

√ see also Stage I, Personal care and hygiene, foot care

√ put out footstool, about 20 cm (8 inches) high

√ in the event of serious pain or malformation of the feet, consult the doctor

Attitude

√ realize that walking remains intact into stage IV of the disease as long as the feet are intact. Good foot care is therefore essential

What the patient can do himself	√ fill a glass with water √ put toothpaste from the tube onto the toothbrush √ clean his teeth with the toothbrush √ take his dentures in and out of his mouth and clean them √ indicate pain in his mouth √ on request: breathe deeply in and out: open and shut his mouth; keep his mouth open; put out his tongue; swallow; bite; chew; suck; spit out; blow

Remind and encourage patient to if necessary explain step by step	√ clean his teeth three times a day; if necessary instruct him to:
	  . "pick up that glass – put some water in it"
	  . "pick up that tube – squeeze it – onto the brush"
	  . "brush – above – below – inside/outside of teeth" (if used to it, also the tongue)
	  . "rinse – with water – spit out"
	  . wipe off – mouth"
	  . "rinse – brush"
	  . in the event of bringing up mucus, spit into a receptacle or facial tissue

Intervene observe for and if necessary prevent	√ not regularly having dentures in the mouth (this leads to getting out of the habit and to rejection of the dentures). This can result in:
	  . avoiding or refusing certain nutriments
	  . not being able to chew and digest properly, leading to inadequate absorption of nourishment, gastrointestinal complaints and difficult bowel movements, and resulting in weight loss
	  . atrophy of the jaw, whereby the dentures no longer fit
	  . pain in the joints of the jaws, which can mimic
	  . earache
	  . speech which is difficult to understand
	  . an 'old' and less recognisable appearance
	√ badly fitting dentures (which do not stay in place; this may cause damage to and infections of the tongue, oral cavity and lips, and difficulties and pain with swallowing

**Partial
take-over**

√ see Stage I, Personal care & hygiene, oral and dental care
√ clean the dentures daily
√ accompany him to the mirror and point out remains of
  food between the teeth and in the corners of the mouth
  and remove them
√ put within reach or give him the requisites for dental
  and oral care. He often fails to recognize his own
  toothbrush and does not know which tube contains the
  toothpaste
√ clean the toothbrush

**Total
take-over**

√ after cleaning the dentures put them into fluid for
  the night (whenever customary)
√ in order to avoid breaking the dentures, half fill the
  washbasin with water when taking out and cleaning the
  dentures
√ give soft, non-sticky food (not ground food). Make
  chewing easier by cutting solid food into small pieces

Attitude

√ realize that daily routine actions can usually be carried
  out by the patient when he is encouraged to do so and
  when the necessary toilet requisites are put within his
  reach. It is usually not yet necessary to take over routine
  actions from the patient

What the patient can do himself

√ recognize, name and point to in himself and in another person: head, hair, forehead, eyebrows, eyelashes, left and right eye, nose, mouth, lips, tongue, chin, cheeks and facial wrinkles

√ recognize himself in the mirror

√ distinguish from a group of five toilet requisites: a comb, a hairbrush, a bar of soap, shaver and razor blades

√ wash and dry hair, face, neck and ears.

√ apply soap, shaving cream, skin cream to face and lips

√ shave himself

√ comb his hair or beard

√ blow his nose

Remind and encourage patient to
if necessary
explain
step by step

√ look in the mirror

√ wash his face, ears and neck

√ wash his hair with shampoo, rinse well and rinse a second time

√ apply skin cream from a tube or pot to the cheeks and forehead and rub it in

√ "take that lipstick – look in the mirror – put it on your lips"

√ "take that comb – look in the mirror – comb your hair"

√ "take that shaving cream – put it on your face"

√ "take that shaver – shave"

√ "take that tissue – blow your nose"

Intervene
observe for
and if neces-
sary prevent
or address

√ see also Stage I, Personal care and hygiene, facial care

√ problems with finding words: he recognizes the toilet article and knows what it is for, but may not be able to name it

√ right use of cream: he often does not know what is in which tube or pot and what it is for

√ soap in the eyes, which can cause panic and falling

√ the accomplishment of a task: in order to get an action going it is sometimes only necessary to hand him the required article; the action is then often completed automatically

**Partial
take-over**

√ see also Stage I, Personal care and hygiene, facial care
√ when several cosmetics are being used, give the patient
the appropriate tube or pot without cap or lid
√ measure out shampoo into his hand or if necessary put
onto his head
√ completion of make-up
√ make a parting and brush/comb hair into shape
√ if necessary, shave off parts of beard which have been
missed out, or trim beard and mustache

**Total
take-over**

√ see also Stage I, Personal care and hygiene, facial care
√ put necessary toilet requisites out clearly and within his
reach
√ only let him use his own shaver with which he is
familiar
√ see that the razor blades are regularly replaced in the
shaver or that the electric shaver is in good condition
√ staunch bleeding from razor nicks with a styptic pencil
√ disinfect small facial wounds with disinfectant
√ see that he has a clean facial tissue with him

Attitude

√ realize that apparent indifference to how one looks is
probably due to loss of initiative and powerlessness.
Neglecting one's appearance often leads to the patient
being less respectfully approached by other people

What the patient can do himself	√ choose from underwear and outerwear if the choice is limited to no more than two items
	√ name most items of clothing
	√ take clothes out of the closet and lay or hang them in the closet
	√ indicate the choice with regard to what he does or does not want to put on
	√ orientate the items of clothing to his own body with regard to right/left, top/bottom, in front/at the back and above/below
	√ perform all the habitual actions as described in chapter 2: stage I, clothing, column 1, item 9
	√ put on all items of clothing by himself with the exception of belt, tie, suspenders
	√ use most standard fastenings: buttons, zippers, snap fasteners, velcro
	√ put on watch, bracelet, earrings or necklace
	√ put personal belongings into handbag/wrist bag and take them out
Remind and encourage patient to if necessary explain step by step	√ take his clothes out of the closet before beginning to dress
	√ begin and continue to get dressed
	√ get dressed sitting down
	√ (for women) wear a bra
	√ pull clothes into position correctly, do up fastenings
	√ fasten necklace, bracelet, earrings
	√ after dressing look in the mirror
	√ put necessary items into handbag/wrist bag, e.g. facial tissue, comb, purse
Intervene observe for and if necessary prevent	√ frustration, agitation, fear, wobbling and inclination to fall when dressing
	√ mime and gestures which indicate feelings of discomfort
	√ badly fitting clothes if the caregiver tidies clothing on the patient's body without asking his permission, this can sometimes lead to anger and agression, since the patient feels his independence is being encroached on)
	√ welts, itching, raw patches or blisters on the skin due to too tight or wrinkling clothes

Partial take-over	√ see also chapter 2: stage I, Partial take-over
	√ accompany patient to closet or wardrobe
	√ help him choose his clothes in the right order and let him lay them out in this order or put them out for him in the right order
	√ if necessary do up shoe laces
	√ do his tie for him
	√ do up or undo belt or suspenders
	√ close all fastenings correctly
	√ straighten out folds and wrinkles in tights or sleeves
	√ assist him with putting his clothes away after undressing
Total take-over	√ reduce underwear to two items on the shelf
	√ determine combinations and variations of outer wear suitable to the season and hang not more than two items of each in his closet for him to choose from
	√ change the two items of clothing daily and out of sight of the patient
	√ clean his shoes – check soles and heels
	√ check clothing for spots, holes or splits
	√ comfortable room temperature
	√ regularly check to what extent the goal of being able 'to dress oneself independently' can be attained
	√ if necessary split the task of dressing himself up into component actions (see chapter 4: stage B: **Clothing**)
	√ wear identification bracelet
Attitude	√ accept the fact that the patient does nothing on his own initiative
	√ let him do what he is able to do himself
	√ if necessary, casually complete the dressing procedure, do not make reproaches when he does not dress correctly
	√ proceed from one action to another in an orderly manner and not too hastily. Taking hold of the patient unexpectedly or roughly causes heightened muscular tension and defensive reactions
	√ see that the patient does not wear nightclothes during the day and vice versa

What the
patient can
do himself

√ go and sit at the table if invited or requested
√ eat with a knife and fork
√ butter a slice of bread or roll and cut it, prepare a
   simple sandwich
√ cut tender meat or fish, without bones
√ move and pick up food with a metal fork
√ if a bowl is passed to him, dish up solid and liquid food
   with a spoon
√ put a spoonful of liquid food into his mouth without
   spilling
√ use cutlery to eat from a plate without moving the plate
   or spilling food over the edge
√ shake out of a pack, e.g. cornflakes
√ at the table take what he wants to eat
√ drink out of a cup, mug and glass without spilling
√ suck up a drink through a drinking straw
√ put food in his mouth with his fingers
√ lick up food with his tongue
√ indicate when food and drink are too hot or too cold
√ use a table napkin to wipe his mouth, chin and fingers
   during the meal
√ indicate thirst and hunger
√ go to the cupboard or refrigerator to help himself to
   something to eat or drink if hungry or thirsty
√ on request put plates, cups and saucers on the table

Remind and
encourage
patient to
if necessary
explain
step by step

√ go to the toilet before the meal
√ wear his dentures
√ take his place at the table
√ if he wears glasses: to put them on during the meal
√ drink enough during the meal
√ eat more slowly or to continue eating when necessary
√ chew thoroughly before swallowing when necessary
√ if all the courses are put out on a tray at the same time,
   eat them in the right order
√ wipe off his mouth, chin and fingers with the table
   napkin after the meal

Intervene
observe for
and if neces-
sary prevent

√ factors interfering with the appetite such as:
. fear, restlessness, apathy
. lack of physical exercise during the day and
   lack of fresh air
. unfriendly atmosphere
. boredom, monotony, sadness,isolation, eating alone
. lack of variety in meals
. badly fitting dentures, not wearing one's dentures
. dry mouth, caused by presence of less saliva or certain
   medicines
. problems with swallowing (such as for example
   caused by sore throat or toothache)
. loss of smell and taste
. conditions such as: inflammation of the mouth,
   cystitis, diarrhea, pneumonia, fever
. constipation
√ usage of correct quantities of seasoning or sugar
√ serving out too large portions
√ cutting with the blunt side of the knife, which causes
   the food to slip off the plate

**Partial
take-over**

√ pass the dishes during the meal

Total
take-over

√ see to nutritious and varied meals
√ total preparation of the meals
√ throw away tainted food
√ lay the table
√ aperitif before and a glass of wine with the meal if the patient is used to it
√ take dishes, crockery, cutlery off the tray and put food and drink within his reach
√ pour water or beverage out in a glass
√ take bones out of meat or fish
√ provide a clean napkin
√ see that there is a restful atmosphere without distraction during the meal
√ in the event of persistent lack of appetite or loss of weight, consult the doctor
√ provide a nonslip table mat to prevent his plate from slipping away

Attitude

√ realize that eating habits can change drastically such as:
  . table manners
  . liking or distaste for certain food
  . lack of appetite or abnormal appetite
√ allow the patient sufficient time to eat
√ involve him in the table conversation
√ do not reproach him or grumble if something goes wrong during the meal
√ take account of the fact that he:
  . wants to sit close to someone he likes
  . cannot talk and eat simultaneously, must concentrate fully on what he is doing
  . is sensitive to the atmosphere at table

What the patient can do himself

√ go to the toilet when he is aware of the urge or when his stomach feels uncomfortable
√ put the light on in his own toilet
√ lock the toilet door behind him
√ urinate standing up
√ sit down, and stand up from the toilet seat
√ when seated grasp toilet paper within his reach
√ wipe himself clean with toilet paper after evacuation
√ throw the used toilet paper in the toilet bowl
√ flush the toilet after using it
√ see to clothes before and after going to the toilet
√ after performing the necessary actions unlock and open the door, turn off the light and close the door behind him
√ indicate and pinpoint discomfort in the private parts and anus

Remind and encourage patient to
if necessary explain step by step

√ go to the toilet at set times and at regular intervals
√ pull clothing up or down and open properly
√ wipe himself off well
√ flush the toilet after use
√ see that clothes are in order
√ turn off the light and close the door after using the toilet
√ go to the toilet in the evening before going to bed
√ urinate before leaving the house for any length of time

Intervene
observe for, and assist when

√ getting lost on the way to the toilet
√ signs of the urge to go to the toilet such as:
. getting restless
. nervously rubbing his arms or legs
. becoming very talkative or very silent
. touching the private parts
. pulling up her skirt or pulling it tightly down over the knees
. continually pressing the knees together

Intervene	√ complaints or signs of pain when urinating or passing a motion. This may cause anxiety about going to the toilet

√ constipation or diarrhea

√ bloodstains on the underpants which may indicate bleeding piles or scratches from itching

outside his own home:
  . signs of the urge to go to the toilet
  . putting clothes in order after going to the toilet

Partial take-over

√ if necessary switch on the light in the toilet

√ if necessary adjust clothing for patient when sitting on toilet

√ if necessary put clothes in order after the visit to the toilet

√ to promote regular motions, accompany him to the toilet shortly after breakfast

√ accompany patient to the toilet in good time after he has taken diuretics. The urge to urinate comes up more rapidly with certain diuretics

√ in the event of restlessness in the night accompany him to the toilet

outside his own home:
  . accompany him to the toilet
  . turn toilet light on and off
  . inspect toilet seat and toilet paper
  . prevent locking of toilet door by the patient
  . wait for the patient outside the toilet
  . if necessary, flush toilet
  . if necessary, put patient's clothes in order
  . operate faucet and hand-drier, or indicate hand towel, if necessary

Total take-over

√ always prevent the toilet door being locked from inside by the patient

√ supervision of hygiene connected with visit to toilet

√ see that breakfast consists of bread rich in fiber, and adequate amounts of liquids

√ see that there is adequate light to find the toilet at night

√ clean and treat piles or sore places in the anal cleft or groin

√ visit the doctor in the event of persisting discomfort (see also stage I, **Personal care, going to the toilet**)

√ choose a place in a restaurant or other public place from which the toilet can be reached quickly and easily

√ if the patient frequently gets lost on the way to the toilet, a clearly visible line placed on the floor leading to the toilet and marking the toilet door may be helpful

Attitude

√ realize that if accidental loss of urine or feces occurs in stage II, the cause probably lies in concomitant factors which can be dealt with (such as a bladder infection or diabetes) and that it is not the result of the dementia process

CHAPTER 4

PARTIAL TAKE-OVER

This is the most difficult stage, both for the patient and also for the caregiver, as it is in this phase that general disorganization of the personality occurs. The changes which take place are now clearly evident to strangers. In the space of about two and a half to three years the patient's level of functioning drops from that of a five-year-old child to that of a child of about two years old. Through the loss of language the patient can no longer adequately put his emotions and experiences into words. The performance of the daily routine activities, such as washing and dressing, already learnt in childhood and carried out more or less automatically ever since, now poses problems and has to be taken over by the caregiver to an increasing extent. During the last part of this stage even the awareness of control of the call of nature is entirely lost. The motor functions now also become visibly disturbed. This rapid disintegration of the mental faculties and of the patient's functioning in general, which causes a complete loss of his independence, is often accompanied by serious behavioral disturbances. The almost total incapacitation, in combination with serious behavioral disturbances, often leads later in this stage to the patient being admitted to a nursing home.

In the course of this stage the patient becomes more and more disoriented with regard to the notion of time and space. He is scarcely conscious of what is going on outside his own immediate environment. He is no longer sure of where he lives and is often unable to give his address. He does not really "live" anywhere anymore, he is passively staying somewhere in a more or less familiar place. He experiences everything going on in his immediate surroundings as random incidents, isolated and unconnected, out of the blue. When he is indoors, he has no conception of outside. He has no idea of what has preceded the moment of here and now and keeps asking in surprise: "How did I get here?" "What am I doing here?" 'Here" is the only thing he is aware of – there is no yesterday and no tomorrow; at best there is a vague notion of "some other time", "not now". He no longer has any idea of the year, month, season or day of the week and sometimes not even of day or night. He gets up in the middle of the night, gets dressed and wanders about the house. In his own home he still knows the way, but in the nursing home he has difficulty in finding his own room and goes into somebody else's, which sometimes upsets the occupant.

His personal past also becomes increasingly blurred; he usually still remembers where he was born and what sort of work he used to do. The reservoir of memories on which he can draw becomes emptier all the time. Relapses into the past occur; the patient is convinced he is still on his job, or is back at home with his parents. Occasionally, repressed emotional events from the past are vividly re-experienced as though they are taking place here and now. Thus, for instance, a patient in a nursing home had frightening hallucinations in which she very vividly re-experienced what had happened to her when she was inprisoned in a camp during the war, and she begged the nursing staff not to torture her in the language of her former captors.

Perceptions can now become disconnected and chaotic. The patient sometimes gets confused when someone speaks to him, because he is unable to locate or link the sound impressions of the speaker's voice with the speaker's face. While he is standing opposite his partner, he asks: "Where are you?" and looks in the wrong direction.

He can still distinguish familiar faces from those of people unknown to him, and he recognizes his children if they visit him regularly, but he no longer knows their names. His marriage partner and his regular caregiver remain familiar to him, although he may sometimes forget their names and confuse their actual identity. His own face often shows bewilderment.

He is very appreciative of compliments and rewards these by telling the person who paid him a compliment, that he is very fond of him and that the latter looks so nice and friendly. These remarks are sometimes accompanied by the request: "May I give you a kiss?" A friendly word or gesture seldom fails to have an effect, as in the case of a very silent patient, who had not spoken any more for months, ever since he was admitted to a nursing home. When a newly arrived caregiver complimented him on how dashing he looked, he went up to her and gently kissed her on the forehead.

On the other hand the patient is also very vulnerable to unkind words and gestures, in particular when he experiences these as disapproval and rejection. Thus a patient began to cry uncontrollably when her daughter told the doctor in her presence about the problems which she sometimes had in looking after her mother. The patient interpreted this as criticism of her behavior. She complained that her daughter no longer loved her, that she felt worthless and wanted to die. When the daughter thereupon burst into tears, the mother put her arm round her daughter and said: "But I love you, you know I do."

Patients in this stage of the illness are often aware that they are a burden to others. That leads to fear of being left in the lurch and sent to a nursing home. The patient realizes that he is totally dependent on the caregiver and is he sometimes frightened of being alone, even for a moment. He keeps following the caregiver about, as though he were attached to him with a rope.

It now becomes difficult to have a conversation with the patient. He can only express himself in short stereotype sentences. He can sometimes give a short answer to simple questions, but he often fails to understand what the other person is saying. His answers are often incoherent and may consist of direct associations with what he observes in his environment or what he feels intensely at that particular moment. A patient who was asked how she felt, looked intently at the floor, picked up a piece of fluff and said: "Someone is not doing her work properly here." Another patient, who was asked by the doctor if he still had his own teeth, answered: "My teeth are chattering"; he was feeling cold. Patients with dentures take the doctor's request to show him their teeth literally and take their dentures out of their mouth, and they comment: "these are not mine".

Some patients talk nonstop incoherently, once they have got into their stride, or they repeat every question which is asked verbatim.

The motor functions undergo clearly visible changes in this stage. Movements gradually cease to be purposeful; the patient can no longer determine the goal of his movements and he keeps losing sight of it. The movements, which in themselves are still intact, thereby acquire a somewhat mechanical and wooden quality and become hesitant and searching in character. When the patient walks, he takes smaller steps and his arms no longer move. But he can still walk faster and swing his arms on request. His facial expression is sometimes void and staring. He no longer looks around him and takes an interest in things, unless he is stimulated by another person. Periods of passivity alternate with periods in which there is a greatly increased, but purposeless urge to move, which manifests itself as general restlessness. The patient may keep on trying to run away, to leave the house, and if he succeeds, he is unable to find his way home again. He also may spend hours pacing up and down in the house, even at night. Sometimes he empties cupboards and drawers, piles up the objects he has taken out and tries to put them back again, usually in the wrong place. Or he keeps on folding up clothes or hand towels and putting them in piles. If the caregiver brusquely tries to stop him from doing these activities, he can get furious. The kinetic energy can then turn into agression. That sometimes leads to shrieking, banging on the door, kicking and hitting. The anger aroused can sometimes be directed in all its violence against the unsuspecting caregiver. Fortunately these fits of anger do not usually last very long and cease as soon as the patient is left alone. In general, his anger is aroused by frustration. In many cases the cause of the frustration can be determined and avoided.

In the course of this stage of the illness, which can be devided into two phases, the patient becomes just as helpless and dependent on the caregiver as a two-year-old child. During the first phase (Stage III A), he successively can no longer wash and dress himself alone and go to the toilet independently. During the second phase, (Stage III B) he can no longer keep his bladder and bowel movement under control. First come the difficulties with dressing himself. Some patients put their clothes on over their pajamas. Others have great problems with the constantly changing form of the garment and cannot get any grip on it when they try to put it on. They lose sight of their 'dressing scheme'; that is, the totality of the principle and the procedures which together constitute the action of dressing oneself. They come to a halt halfway if they get stuck on one particular detail. A piece of fluff on their skirt or trousers can compulsively absorb their attention, preventing them from getting any further.

Apart from difficulties with the 'dressing scheme' and the handling of clothes, the patient is now and again confused with regard to his own body. He has problems with notions such as right and left, in front and behind, above and below. Subsequently he loses the notion of how the different parts of the body are related to the body as a whole, and finally he becomes totally oblivious to the fact that he has a body.

Difficulties occur next with bathing and showering, which he then can no longer do independently. Choosing between two faucets and adjusting them to regulate the temperature of the water becomes impossible. The sudden cascading of the shower water sometimes alarms and disorientates him and he may experience difficulty in maintaining his balance. All this can turn the daily washing session into a real trial. While he is being washed by someone else, he may not know whether the actions are being carried out by his own hand or by that of the caregiver. It is sometimes impossible for him to link tactile sensations and visual impressions any longer. It can happen that the patient tries to copy every movement of the caregiver's, as though the latter were his mirror image. All this is another sign of the beginning of the loss of the body scheme, i.e. the orientation towards one's own body.

In this stage most patients can still recognize themselves in the mirror. But if they are are not able to see themselves in the mirror every day, a sudden confrontation with their own face can be a shocking experience. This was, for example, the case with an eighty-year-old demented woman, who had previously been a well-known actress. In the nursing home she was visited by a doctor and a nurse. Much of her conversation was incoherent and it was difficult for her to comprehend simple questions. She had surrounded herself with photos of herself taken in bygone years, which she always carried about and proudly showed to visitors. When the doctor held a mirror in front of her to see whether she still recognized herself, she groaned and knocked the mirror out of his hand. When the mirror was again held up in front of her, she called out, filled with aversion: "No, no", picked up one of her close-up photos and held it in front of her face. That was who she was, not the scared old face in the mirror.

Towards the end of this third stage patients often fail to recognize their own mirror image any more and think there is a stranger in the room, when they see themselves in the mirror. They may talk to their mirror image, and sometimes they get angry with the 'stranger'. Another patient said on seeing his mirror image: "Give him something to eat, he is my friend."

About six months after the difficulties with bathing and showering have begun, the patient can no longer perform the actions involved in going to the toilet without help. He may not wipe himself, throw the toilet paper into the washbasin or fail to use it at all. He may no longer wash his hands after he has finished. He may no longer flush the toilet.

It is now about eighteen months ago that the patient had his first problems with getting dressed. Now he enters the second phase of stage III in which he loses the power of controlling his bladder and bowel movements, because he is incapable of taking the necessary measures when he feels an urge. Initially he may still be aware of his incontinence and it makes him feel ashamed. Sometimes he hides his undershorts away. But gradually he loses all awareness of the moments at which he relieves himself. However, if the caregiver takes him to the toilet at regular intervals, then that can often help to avoid the patient soiling himself for quite a long time.

During this stage, most patients can still feed themselves using a fork and spoon, and can drink from a cup, glass or mug. However, using a knife soon presents problems. Somebody else must cut the meat, get meat off the bone or take bones out of fish. Drinking presents little difficulty, but the patient soon becomes incapable of pouring out liquids. He also needs repeated encouragement to go on with the meal and not to leave the table. Some patients undergo a change in their preference for certain food. The appetite itself usually remains good and is sometimes difficult to satisfy. Nevertheless the patient's weight does often decrease. In some patients chewing begins to slow down.

This stage of partial take-over can make the utmost demands on the caregiver. On account of the dramatic disintegration of his personality, the patient is emotionally very unstable. Behavioral disturbances occur more frequently in this stage than in any other stage. The patient has now increasingly less adequate means at his disposal to express his feelings, needs and urges. Delusions, suspicions and verbal expressions of anxiety are gradually replaced by less well differentiated modes of behavior, such as hallucinations, during which the patient often sees deceased relatives, or episodes of crying without words.

The motor system is still largely intact in this stage, and it is in particular increased and seemingly purposeless motor activity which now prevails. Wandering away, incessantly pacing up and down, incessant querying, lamenting or wailing, opening and closing of doors, drawers or closets, and taking the contents out and putting them back again are all ways in which he tries to channel his energy. The patient often acts with great perseverance and compulsion and attempts to restrain him are often met with anger and sometimes with agression. Apparently unmotivated resistance to suggestions or orders coming from the caregiver occurs not infrequently and may interfere with functioning. This resistance, or negativism, and agression, either verbal or physical, occur in situations of interaction with another person, usually the caregiver. These may be attempts to protect one's ever more vulnerable disintegrating individuality. This requires a lot of patience and understanding from the caregiver. Behavioral disturbances interfere significantly with the patient's functionality. They are sometimes preventable or treatable.

The patient is increasingly at the mercy of his environment to which he is increasingly incapable of adapting. Although his insight into his own situation has greatly diminished, he is nevertheless often painfully confronted with his deterioration, precisely in the interaction with another person. He is continually in the process of parting with more of himself.

The behavior, which the outside world observes, gives some indication of the way in which each individual patient copes with this disease, which is slowly but surely robbing him of his world. Each patient does this with the means at his disposal. Some patients retain considerable social skills and retain a remarkable sense of humor. They remain oriented to contact with another person and pay that person compliments as a sign of their appreciation of his interest in them. In a sense these patients function better and have fewer problems with the care giver because they are so friendly and compliant. Other patients withdraw into their shell and reject all contact, or are easily angered and resist all help. Each patient tries in his own way to defend and maintain his individuality as much and as long as possible. If the caregiver recognizes that and empathizes, much of the disturbed behavior will become more comprehensible and manageable.

Certain forms of disturbed behavior, such as refusal or resistance, frequently interfere with the caregiver's attempts to assist the patient in his daily personal care. Much tact and patience are required. It sometimes helps to overcome the patient's resistance if the caregiver, whenever feasable, performs the same activity on himself, together with the patient. In some cases, however, psychoactive medication is required to control behavior which is harmful to the patient or his environment.

The functions of personal care, which are subsequently lost in this stage, are heavily invested with cultural and social values. The patient does not merely lose particular functions. It is the relevance which these actions have for him that is completely lost out of his sight. There is not only a loss of memory, or a loss of praxis. There is the loss of the brain mechanisms which are the foundation of social behavior. At the end of this stage the patient has lost to a considerable extent the ability of active social interaction with other persons.

Caring for and nursing persons with dementia is more than a question of technical actions. Everyone who is involved with these people knows how even the most demented person is sensitive to an attitude of kindness and deference. Many a visitor in a nursing home has had the experience in which the patient looks at him with enquiring eyes and begs him either in words or by gripping his hand: "Please don't go away."

What the patient can do himself

√ take part in selected outdoor activities together with a healthy partner, such as

√ water or pick flowers in the garden, use a watering can, rake up leaves, push a light wheelbarrow, carry and pile logs

√ help wash the car

√ feed animals in the zoo or at the farm

√ push a baby carriage/buggy

√ push or pull a shopping cart

√ sit at the water's edge and feed ducks

√ walk along even trails in the outdoors or along the beach

√ paddle on the beach or in shallow water

√ sit quietly outside in the garden, in the country or on the porch

Remind and encourage patient to

√ wear his glasses and a hearing aid. Seeing clearly and hearing the human voice and the sound of nature promote his continuing contact with the environment

Intervene observe for, and if necessary prevent

√ contractures of the joints which cause premature loss of ambulation: permanent malformation and contracture of joints soon occur if long periods are passively spent in a wheelchair. In this connection heightened muscular tension, which is often prominent in this stage of the disease, and changes related to aging are factors which greatly increase the risk. Contractures can occur in all the joints. Once deformity of the joints has occurred, the damage cannot be repaired. The occurrence of contractures can in this stage be avoided by letting the patient take part as long as possible in the activities of personal care and hygiene and by means of various recreational activities which promote movement of all joints

√ wandering away from the garden – he usually does not recognize his own garden any more

√ protect him from overexposure to the heat of the sun in the summer and from cold in the winter

Partial take-over

√ outdoors and indoors direct his vision by indicating a particular object in space and saying: "Look, there is..." This temporarily widens his world and directs his attention, and may cause him to walk faster.

√ encourage him to accompany you for a walk by setting a specific goal: i.e., gather acorns, shells, flowers etc., feed the ducks or walk the dog

√ when outdoors always supervise and guide the patient

Total take-over

√ fit daily locomotor and psychomotor recreational activities into the weekly scheme of activities.

Note: Guided locomotor and psychomotor activities are an important means of structurizing the patient's energies in this stage. In addition, these activities may promote:

– stimulation of the motor functions
– oriented use of the senses
– working off energy, tension and fear
– contact with the surrounding world
– exercising muscles and joints in order to prevent stiffness, avoid contractures and decubitus, and maintain general daily physical functions
– physical fatigue which may result in sleeping better at night
– prevention of constipation
– improvement of the blood circulation
– increased appetite
– stimulation of head movements, which may help to prevent a permanent stiffening of the neck
– stimulation of arm movements, preventing the arms from becoming continually turned inwards and pressed against the body or held away from the body
– stimulation of hand and finger movements, preventing the wrists from becoming permanently turned in the direction of the thumbs, and the finger tips from pressing into the palm of the hand
– stimulation of trunk movements, as a result of which the spinal column does not become permanently arched forward or sideways

    — stimulation of shoulder and hip movements, preventing
these joints from becoming permanently flexed and
turned inwards

    — stimulation of foot movements, preventing the ankle
joints from stiffening and the Achilles tendon from
shortening

Attitude   √ create an environment in which the patient can live
with as much freedom of movement as possible. The
wheelchair, in which in the middle of stage III he is
often compelled to spend large parts of the day in
idleness, while he can still walk independently,
represents a punishment for him. One of the last
possible ways of physical interaction with his
environment is then prematurely lost. What is left to
him then is only banging or screaming

What the patient can do himself

√ together with a healthy partner take part in a variety of indoor activities such as:
. drawing, coloring, painting
. tearing and crumpling paper
. sticking things on paper or cardboard
. clay modeling
. arranging flowers
. arranging things sort by sort
. picking out things that feel the same
. putting things away and turning things out
. fitting together construction components with divergent forms
. doing simple jigsaw puzzles
. matching up identical figures and colors
. hail and farewell game (see next page)
. playing a musical instrument and singing
. walking in a structured space
. (square) dancing
. playing with a ball, rope or hoop

Intervene observe for, and if necessary prevent

√ frustration or anger. Not every person enjoys the same activities. If the patient indicates that he does not like a particular activity or has had enough of it, he should not be compelled to continue
√ unsafe use of materials by the patient

Attitude

√ realize that regular shifts of the body posture and physical activity are of great importance. In the late part of this stage in particular, the patient often no longer knows how to get his body into a comfortable position while seated in a chair for longer periods of time. Shouting and restlessness may indicate that his body is in an uncomfortable and painful position. Prolonged inactivity in the sitting position slowly forces the body into permanently assuming the form of sitting posture in the chair, which can eventually result in the patient being unable to lie stretched out and on his back in bed

What the patient can do himself

√ say goodbye. Comprehend the action of parting, whereby one person leaves the other, and make farewell gestures:
. shake a hand extended to him
. give a kiss on an offered cheek, hand or mouth
. wave in response as a sign of greeting

√ repeat words and sentences like:
. bye! hello! hi!
. see you in a minute
. see you soon
. so long

√ recognize words and gestures as friendly or unfriendly

√ become attached to, and maintain emotional contact with someone kindly inclined to him

√ resist contact with someone whom he experiences as unfriendly and obtrusive

Remind and encourage patient to

√ respond to a greeting

Intervene observe for, and if necessary prevent

√ the words 'see you soon', 'so long' are notions relating to a period in the future. Because of the loss of the concept of time and space, going away means being gone and not coming back. The patient lives in the here and now, gone is gone. Only the other person's physical presence is guarantee of his being available to the patient. He is unable to anticipate a reunion in in the future. An acute feeling of anxiety may occur in such a situation, which is experienced as a sudden loss. This may be accompanied by a feeling of abandonment and great uncertainty

Total take-over

√ try to provide a feeling of security with regard to meeting again after parting

√ hail and farewell by means of a game:

1 a few times a day the caregiver casually goes out of the room and then enters the room again, saying, for example, "Hello!" or "There I am again!"

2 as a surprise let some possession of the patient's disappear and reappear, by covering it over for a moment, keeping it in your hand or putting it in the trouser pocket

3 exchange: swap similar personal objects, such as one another's wristwatch, pocket comb, ring, jacket, coat, shoe. Method: sit down opposite the patient and take the initiative. The caregiver puts an object in front of him or first gives something himself and then says: "Give me your..." After a pause he says: "May I have... back." If necessary he points to the object in question

Attitude

√ try to identify with the patient in his fear of parting. Purely verbal assurance of coming back is insufficient and not understood by the patient

√ realize that the feeling of being physically 'together' is very important for the patient. This is in particular true for this stage, where the patient experiences an overwhelming feeling of helplessness. The being there of another person also enforces his own feeling of being there. The patient forms an entity with the caregiver, from whom he can no longer detach himself. Losing his caregiver means losing himself.

This also causes a feeling of being abandoned and of losing the other's affection

What the patient can do himself	√ with difficulty carry on a conversation using simple words in the language of his own social and cultural milieu √ perform stereotype repetitive patterns of movement √ distinguish the colors red, yellow, blue and green and sometimes name them √ match up identical pictures and sheets of color, pick them up; hold them; look at them; compare them; put next to or on top of each other
Remind and encourage patient to explain each step because he no longer knows the right order; before encouraging him, call him by his name	√ practice matching by demonstration and imitatation, demonstrate, let him imitate and indicate. First direct his attention to the object: "Just look at this..." or "There is...". Then, after a short pause, repeat in a friendly voice: "Pick ... up, put ... down". The patient's actions are often no longer directed to the goal, but consist mainly of sensory reconnaissance of the objects brought to his attention, by looking, feeling and searching
Intervene observe for, and if necessary prevent	√ the conversations of the Alzheimer patients among themselves become increasingly a one-way communication; there is little attention to one another √ because he is increasingly incapable of making his wishes and displeasure known, he becomes more vulnerable and less tolerant and can be subject to abrupt changes of mood √ he no longer understands the notion of doing something 'in turn' with another person √ he quickly loses interest if the exercise is not continued or if he is constantly corrected √ the notions of 'mine and thine' are lost

Partial take-over	√ utilize his stereotype, single repetitive movements by means of objects. This structurizes the movement and has a stimulating and calming effect on the patient √ let the game proceed spontaneously and observe what happens √ avoid sudden and unexpected movements

Total take-over	√ choose a suitable game, consisting of single repetitive movements, and put it out ready
	√ materials for matching up identical pictures:
	  - a frame, 12 x 6 inches or 24 x 16 cm, with compartments for 6 pictures, 4 x 2 inches or 8 x 8 cm each
	  - two copies of colored pictures with a particular theme, for instance personal care: a face, hand, comb, toothbrush, bath, toilet; bedroom or sitting room furniture
	√ materials for matching up identical colors:
	  - make a frame, 8 x 8 inches (20 x 20 cm), divided into 4 compartments
	  - make two copies each of color sheets in red, yellow, green and blue

Attitude	√ allow him to act in a playful way √ face up to the fact that during stage III the patient becomes 'blind with his eyes open and deaf with his ears open'. His ability to recognize objects becomes increasingly impaired. Consequently they become meaningless to him. He becomes increasingly incapable of contact at a distance via looking and listening. He cannot anticipate anymore. Everything seems to happen unexpectedly, out of the blue √ recognize and accept an increasingly stereotype behavioral pattern in the patient with a marked involuntary urge to continual repetition of apparently pointless movements or actions

What the   √ do puzzles:
patient can   . by means of trial and error put together the
do himself   pieces of a jigsaw puzzle, consisting of no more than
                       about twenty large pieces which have been taken
                       apart; the jigsaw is surrounded by a frame
                    . fit large figures into a smooth base in which there are
                       sunken impressions of these figures
                  √ fit together and take apart construction components by
                    means of:
                    . screws – wind the nut round the thread
                    . pushing – get pieces to engage by pressing
                    . fit a tongue into a groove, thereby connecting two
                       pieces up into one
                    . allow two pieces to engage one another by means of
                       a coupling
                    . put square or cylindrical forms into appropriate
                       square or round opening and take them out again

Remind and   √ join pieces or components together
encourage   √ praise him when he goes on trying
patient to

Intervene   √ frustration or discouragement
observe for,
and if neces-
sary prevent

Total   √ provide material consisting of large pieces,
take-over   which are easy to manipulate
                  √ put the materials on a nonslip mat to prevent them
                    shifting
                  √ provide materials with holes or hollows, into which
                    other things can be fitted, such as:
                    . an egg rack or box with imitation eggs
                    . a plank with holes in it, through which pipes can be
                       hung or in which plastic test tubes can be placed

Attitude   √ the emphasis is put on stimulation of psychomotor
activity in the patient, together with another person, as
a means of making contact. Curiosity and perseverance
may motivate some patients, while other patients are
simply absorbed in repetitive actions

What the patient can do himself	√ assort according to:
	  . form or category
	  . color
	  . things feeling the same when touched
	√ put the assorted objects:
	  . onto each other
	  . in a row
	  . in a pile
	  . in order of size – from large to small and vice versa
	   examples:
	  . arrange flowers
	  . distinguish their colors and length
	  . indicate what he likes or dislikes
	  . arrange them in his own way in a vase
	  . open and close a box
	  . put objects into it and take them out of it

Intervene observe for, and if necessary prevent	√ frustration or anger because he finds the activity childish √ at the end of this stage III the patient is no longer interested in lifeless objects as such, since he can no longer recognize them and do anything with them. He then principally experiences objects through the sense of touch
Partial take-over	√ put flowers or materials in front of him, so that he can finger them or look at them √ put the materials to be used within his reach, such as a number of already folded kitchen or bath towels; or books with a stiff cover

**Total
take-over**

√ obtain suitable materials, such as for instance
. artificial flowers and an unbreakable vase with a heavy base
. pick only nonpoisonous flowers
. for sorting: acorns, pine cones, shells, small stones, hazel and walnuts
. for putting into and taking out, sorting and transferring, buy two transparent storage pots with necks wide enough to put your hand in easily
. collect a variety of materials that can be put in the pots
. for tactile stimulation collect materials with different texture or form, such as:
   - pieces of fluffy, hairy, rough, smooth or ribbed fabric, 8 by 8 inches (20 by 20 cm)
   - round, square, corrugated or smooth objects such as buttons
. provide a box with a hinged lid, 6 by 3 inches (15 by 7 cm) for opening and shutting, putting in and taking out etc.

Attitude

√ take into account that the individual preference, interest and still remaining concentration vary considerably, whereby the previous history and occupation of the patient can play a role. Materials for activities can be selected accordingly. Children's toys are often rejected as being too childish

What the patient can do himself	√ make music on his own instrument √ recognize the different sounds of certain musical instruments,e.g., piano, recorder, flute, violin, accordion, harmonica, without being able to name them √ indicate which sounds he likes or dislikes √ make rhythmic sounds with his hands; play a percussion instrument rhythmically to the beat of accompanying music √ join in singing simple, familiar songs √ clap his hands and rock his body to and fro
Intervene observe for, and if necessary prevent	√ shrill, penetrating sounds which may arouse negative emotions in the patient and can make him restless, fearful and sometimes agressive.
Partial take-over	√ give him his musical instrument regularly and encourage him to play it √ stimulate him to listen and participate when there are musical events √ give him a good quality percussion instrument and encourage him to produce the sound himself, for example a drum, a gong with an echo, a cowbell
Total take-over	√ see also stage II Music and singing √ sit opposite the patient and sing with him and make accompanying gestures with your hands. Examples: . Old McDonald had a farm . Dickory Dock . Ride a cock-horse . See-saw, Marjorie Daw . When I was a tailor √ invite someone to play and talk about his musical instrument such as a flute, violin or accordeon. A solo performer creates a congenial atmosphere and engages the patient in the performance. This is possible in a group of not more than four patients.

Attitude √ one can experiment with various forms of music and various types of instruments according to what is best suited to the individual patient. Making music together, joining in singing or letting the patient hum has a relaxing and at the same time engaging effect

What the patient can do himself	√ with little control over the finer hand and finger movements: drawing, coloring, water color painting √ use a thick, long brush, pencil or felt-tip on large sheets of paper √ if the patient has had previous experience, he can also choose and work with brushes of different thicknesses, and rinse them each time before using another color. He can then do work with four colors √ as an alternative: work with two colors of watercolor, with one brush for each color Or: one color of paint but brushes of different thicknesses √ work with a maximum of four different crayons: red, yellow, blue and green √ sometimes still draw more or less recognizable figures with a pencil or felt-tip on paper √ distinguish between the colors red, yellow, blue and green and sometimes name them
Encourage patient	√ by proposing to join him in drawing or painting together with him
Intervene observe for, and if necessary prevent	√ working on too small a sheet of paper with too fine a pencil, because the patient lacks the coordinated fine hand and finger movements
Partial take-over	√ offer him the opportunity to find his own form of expression; trying to copy simple examples of drawings in front of him can sometimes help to get him started √ or: together with the patient hold *one* long thick crayon or felt-tip, follow the movements of the patient's hand and see that the crayon stays in contact with the paper. Alternatively, steer the patient's hand over the surface of the paper. Repeat these exercises with different colors.

**Total
take-over**

√ choose materials:
  . non-toxic paint, pencils and felt-tips
  . thick brushes, pencils and felt-tips with long handles
  . large sheets of thick paper, 15 by 22 inches (50 x 50 cm)

√ give him small quantities of oil paint or watercolor to prevent paint dripping off the handle after dipping in

√ fasten the paper down onto a drawing board; shifting paper is discouraging

√ put his name and the date on his drawings and paintings and put them in his own portfolio

Attitude

√ do not ask the patient questions about what his drawing or painting represents. It is a spontaneous production. He is usually incapable of explaining it and repeated querying may irritate him

√ show a genuine interest in his achievement by asking him if he is enjoying it and continually encourage him to express himself in the activity

What the patient can do himself

√ work with modeling clay or dough: knead, press or slap it, bore holes in it with the fingers, cut pieces off and roll and turn it

√ draw and paint from the shoulder and elbow joints (but not from the fingers and wrists)

√ use a thick brush, pencil or felt-tip, with a long handle

√ use a brush of one thickness: dip it in the paint and brush it off on the paper (but do not rinse off in fluid)

√ move a brush with paint, a felt-tip or pencil spontaneously over the paper so that a pattern of lines is produced

√ work with a maximum of two crayons or felt-tips; red and green

Partial take-over

√ give the patient a shapeless piece of clay or dough and take a piece yourself; knead, roll, turn and make holes in it with your finger. This stimulates the patient to copy you. He can sometimes manage to model simple forms such as a doll, ball or worm. Handling clay or dough stimulates the sense of touch, and prompts finger movements and the coordinated use of both hands

What the
patient can
do himself

√ fold out and fold up handicraft materials
√ tear or crumple paper
√ twiddle with objects; restlessly touch something with
   his fingers
√ sort things – by color; by texture; by size
√ paste pieces of paper on paste board

Encourage to √ participate in the activity:
. for instance, by asking him: "Will you tear this paper
   for me?'
. by demonstration: pick up; take out of envelope; tear
   paper; screw paper up into a ball; put down or throw
   into the wastebasket; put paste on paper etc.

Partial
take-over

√ structured tearing and crumpling activity: go
   through the mail with the patient in the morning
√ if possible let the patient take the contents out of the
   envelope, tear the paper, crumple it up and throw into
   the wastebasket
√ let the patient paste the torn and crumpled pieces onto
   a colored background at random, which creates a
   collage

Total
take-over

√ provision of suitable materials:
. envelopes containing junk mail
. sheets of firm, colored background paper 15 by 22
   inches (50 x 50 cm)
. a bulletin board

Attitude

√ handling the mail confronts him with the address
   where he lives and leads to constructive interaction
   between patient and caregiver

What the patient can do himself

√ participate in a round dance or row dance, based on his previous dance experience
√ if taken by his hands, join in a rhythmic motion such as dancing, taking small steps
√ imitate others:
  . make criss-cross movements to the beat of the music
  . get into a circle or row
  . stand still
  . walk hand in hand in the circle
  . walk in a line with the hands on each other's shoulders
  . take one another by the hand
  . put his hands in his waist
  . move arm in arm in a small circle

Encourage patient to

√ imitate the dance movements
√ move to the music with his partner
√ keep his hands in the right place
√ dance with you by saying: "May I dance with you, you are so good at it, can you show me how to do it?" "Shall we try together?"

Intervene observe for, and if necessary prevent

√ walking in a distressed and agitated or searching manner, which can happen when he loses sight of his partner and feels completely lost
√ loss of balance or fearfulness

Partial take-over

√ see Stage II (square) dancing

Total take-over

√ create a secure environment: see Stage II (square)dancing

√ matching of the dance partners. The total number of participants should not exceed six patients and one dance leader

√ see to:
 . going to the toilet or changing the incontinence system before the activity
 . cleaning glasses and letting him wear them
 . adjusting the hearing aid if he wears one
 . well-fitting shoes with nonslip soles and heels and tied shoe laces
 . loosely fitting clothing; check the length of the trouser legs

Attitude

√ exercising to music need not necessarily be dancing, moving to music. It can also be done sitting, standing or even lying down. What matters is: experiencing ones own movement to a rhythm. In dancing, as in every playful exercise, one can get totally involved, purely for the sake of self-movement, free of necessity or pressure. Music and dance invite the patient to participate spontaneously and voluntarily

√ patients suffering from Alzheimer's disease can have a tremendous urge to move. They often respond promptly to an inviting gesture to move

What the patient can do himself

√ change on his own initiative from sitting position to standing, but not always the reverse

√ move from sitting position to standing, remain standing, turn round and walk on

√ when walking lift the sole of the foot from the ground and put down again placing first the forefoot and then the heel (i.e. walking without a heel strike)

√ turn round standing up taking small steps

√ wander; within an unstructured enclosed area walk to and fro restlessly, hesitantly and aimlessly

√ sometimes walk comparatively quickly when stimulated by another person

√ sit quietly for limited periods of time

√ spontaneously but not on command pick up an object by chance, keep hold of it and bring it to an undetermined point

Intervene observe for, and if necessary prevent

√ patient from exhausting himself by pacing:
. in stage III B the patient loses his sense of spatial relations and of the place which his body occupies in space
. when walking, he often allows himself to be guided by certain patterns in the floor covering, such as lines, blocks or flowers, or vertical structures in the wall such as doors

√ uneven floor or terrain which easily causes loss of balance or falling

√ inability to sit down: since he no longer recognizes a chair as a place to sit, he may walk round the chair several times and inspect the seat, not knowing any more how to sit down

√ having his walk interrupted or his path blocked, because that can be experienced as something threatening, which arouses fear and agression in him

√ coming straight towards him or grabbing or pushing him from behind can be experienced as a threat. Advice: approach him obliquely from the side, then stroke his shoulder or back and guide him by the arm to the intended destination

Intervene √ taking hold of the patient or ordering him about
√ if two participants have a disagreement, quietly take the most agitated person's hand, stroke the back of his hand and his back and get him to walk on

**Total
take-over** √ structurize walking by giving it direction and form so that it becomes a more constructive activity, indoors as well as outdoors. Organizational form for six patients:

1 free arrangement of six chairs in a spacious room or on a terrace. Ample space encourages freer movement
2 comfortable straight solid chairs with armrests, in various contrasting colors, which attract the patient's attention
3 arrange the chairs in the walking space and do not move them during the walking period
4 soft music as accompaniment to the movement creates a restful, pleasant atmosphere
5 time the activity to take place as far as possible in accordance with the period of the spontaneous urge to move
6 the supervising person should be familiar with the physical capabilities and behavioral patterns of the participants
7 mark lines, walking patterns on the floor with chalk. Never put loose tiles or other objects on the floor as markers

Attitude √ recognize that the patient is a prisoner in his ever
shrinking world. On his own initiative he is no longer
capable of doing anything else but pace aimlessly. He
continues to fight for the retention of this last remnant
of freedom and he resists restriction of his freedom by
restraints

√ realize that there is a total lack of purpose in his
locomotion. Walking takes place spontaneously from
an inner urge to move

√ give the patients a chance to indulge their inner urge to
move

√ realize that when a patient constantly wants to follow
in the other person's wake, to him this may mean: "The
other person can guide me, I'm lost on my own, alone I
can get nowhere"

What the patient can do himself

√ standing up – throw a ball

√ when seated, catch a ball from close by and throw it back

√ together with a partner: throw the ball across underhand with two hands; pass crosswise; put from one hand into the other; with both hands round the ball, move it forward and back, upwards and downwards; both together with both hands round the same ball – move it backwards and forwards, upwards and downwards, obliquely to the right, obliquely to the left

√ standing or sitting and together with a partner: pull a rope or a hoop to and fro; move it from one hand to the other; let it slide through his hands or trail behind him over the floor

Encourage to demonstrate and let him imitate

√ throw, catch or take hold of ball, rope or hoop

√ pass it from one hand to the other and then pass it over crosswise

√ follow his companion who leads him with the aid of a rope or hoop

√ walk ahead and pull his companion along

Intervene observe for, and prevent

√ loss of equilibrium through bending too far to one side

√ wobbling due to loss of equilibrium or tiredness

Total take-over

√ activate and steer walking activity by:

. casually offering the (circular) rope or a hoop and giving the opportunity to get used to it;

. making slight waving, pulling or pushing movements with the rope or hoop

. walking on, so that he casually and without pressure follows in the direction in which he is being led

√ acquire: foam balls – red, yellow, green and blue, in various sizes, from a tennis ball to a football

√ adjust the pace of the movements to the patient, look out for uneven ground and the presence of objects he might bump into

**What the
patient can
do himself**

From the beginning to the end of stage III he can:
√ walk independently
√ move from lying to sitting to standing position, remain standing, turn round and walk on
√ change: from sitting to standing position and start walking
√ sit upright in a chair unsupported
√ roll over from his stomach to his back and vice-versa
√ lift up his head while lying on his back
√ when lying on his stomach raise his torso leaning on his arms

Intervene
observe for,
and if neces-
sary prevent

√ falling: the risk of a fall becomes ever greater, because the patient becomes gradually unable to assume the necessary posture for the performance of certain actions or he has a constant urge to move
  - he is often unable to remain quietly seated for any length of time
  - subsequently he cannot stand on one foot any more without help
  - thereafter he cannot sit down any more from the walking position on a chair or the edge of a bed without help
  - he cannot go up and down stairs any more
√ not being able to sit down without help at the end of this stage causes him to stand up from the toilet bowl and walk away with his trousers round his knees or ankles. He can move from a lying to a sitting position as he gets out of bed, but he cannot always manage to lie down on the bed again
√ tiredness, aimlessly and fearfully wandering round in a badly lit space soon lead to bumping into things and falls
√ for the patient who uses a walker, the correct order of walking with a walking frame is: first put the frame in front of you, then take two steps, then move the frame again. If the patient can no longer do this, then he should be prevented from using it. In the last phase of this stage he is no longer capable of learning to use the frame independently

Partial take-over

√ movements which make demands on the now disturbed balance reflexes should always be carried out with the patient sitting down for safety

√ move the patient gently and slowly and prevent sudden movement, since he cannot assess what is going to happen and cannot himself determine the pace at which he has to join in the movement. If he is touched unexpectedly, his body stiffens and he becomes frightened, which poses a threat to his equilibrium

√ use a great deal of tact and exercise patience in helping with moving the patient from the standing to the sitting position. His inability to do so may sometimes be interpreted as unwillingness. Letting him dress and undress standing up or denying him his night's rest, because he apparently does not wish to go to bed, may agitate the patient and irritate the caregiver. As a result the patient becomes overtired and can easily have a fall

√ in helping him to sit down, see that the chair does not shift away

√ when he has a tendency to lose his balance when getting out of bed, let him first put on his socks and shoes and put your own foot in front of the patient's foot to prevent slipping

Total take-over

√ prevention of falls:

- by recognizing loss of ambulatory functions in good time

- by stimulation of ambulation through motor recreational pursuits

- avoid prolonged periods of restless sitting and channel the energy and the urge to move by daily alternation of structurized walking, lying and sitting activities

- prevent long periods of aimless and agitated wandering about, which lead to tiredness, stumbling and falling

- avoid long periods of aimlessly sitting in a chair; this leads to agitation and agression, and to falls when he starts to walk again. Muscles and joints become stiff and painful through lack of movement

Total
take-over
- adjust the height of the bed so that when the patient is sitting properly on the bed, the soles of both feet touch the floor. The patient is unable to judge the distance between the bed and the floor
- install a safety gate for the stairs
- at the end of this stage he can no longer walk up and down stairs, get into or out of a bus, tram, train or automobile
- for patients who move about with the aid of a walking frame, the latter should be adjusted in such a way that when the patient leans on it, there is slight bending of the elbows. If the frame is too low, it is pushed forward instead of being lifted, whereby his feet cannot keep pace with his hands. This may cause walking in a stooped position or leaning too much to one side. If the frame is too high, it is difficult to lift it up, which can lead to the patient falling over backwards
- when the patient moves from sitting to standing position,see that he does not pull himself up by the walking frame. He must first push himself up on the armrests of the chair or on the table and only when he is standing, must the frame be placed in front of him. Make sure that he holds the frame firmly and that his standing balance is in order before he starts to walk

Attitude
√ realize that the risk of falling should not result in the patient being forced into unnecessary immobility. This results in the premature loss of the ambulatory functions and may cause screaming

What the patient can do himself	In stage IIIA he can: √ usually recognize, name and point to: head, ears, eyes, nose, mouth, tongue, hair, hands and knees on request √ often distinguish right from left √ engage in a limited simple conversation using single words. Both the vocabulary and the subjects of conversation are very restricted and rambling frequently occurs
Intervene observe for	√ the gradual loss of the ability to recognize, name and point to parts of the body and of the comprehension of how the different parts of the body relate to the whole body. This leads to confusion, perplexity and general helplessness √ in stage IIIB he no longer knows he has a back √ at the end of stage IIIB, he no longer reacts to "Bring your hand to your mouth" or "Point to your nose". He can still instinctively or in a reflex action bring his hand to his mouth. He hears the request, but does not understand it and cannot comply with it. He loses the awareness of his body and its functions
Partial take-over	*body scheme exercises:* - regularly caress and massage all parts of the body - indicate and name parts of the body - devote special attention to the mouth and the hands by demonstrating and imitating movements, such as sticking out your tongue, showing your hand with the fingers stretched or bent or spread out, clenching your fist, etc - practice mime: make funny faces emphasizing the mouth movements and challenge him to imitate you
Total take-over	√ use a doll, the size of a baby, for letting him indicate the parts of the body. In stage III he frequently has to use his sense of touch to confirm what he sees
Attitude	√ continual physical contact confirms the patient in his physicalness √ avoid using the doll in a childish manner

What the patient can do himself

during stage IIIA he can:

√ indicate what he wants and does not want, what he finds pleasant and unpleasant

√ convey feelings of pain

√ move subsequently from lying down to sitting to standing to remaining standing to walking, and backwards

√ undress himself completely on his own

√ if invited get subsequently into the bath or go under the shower, turn round, sit down, and get out or come out of the bath or shower

√ go through the motions of washing and drying his face, arms, chest and stomach, mechanically and with little control of hands and fingers, automatically, more stroking than rubbing

√ put his hand or foot in another person's hand, extended to him

√ hold onto a handrail attached to the wall and pull himself up from the sitting position

Remind and encourage patient to
if necessary explain
step by step

√ wash himself, while in the tub or shower: by means of kind explicit requests accompanied by demonstration, and inviting him to imitate you. First direct his attention to his hand and then to the part of the body to be washed. His actions are no longer oriented to a goal and no longer take place according to a preconceived plan of action. He often does not react to the request: "Wash your face, wash your arm, roll onto your side or point to your leg". He no longer understands a complex request, nor can he carry it out. Irritation with and the rejection of the caregiver may ensue

Intervene
observe for, and if necessary prevent

√ signs of panic: the patient may be afraid of a cold or slippery floor; of water falling on his head; of washing his face and hair; of loss of control over the situation and of being submitted to a procedure the purpose of which escapes him

. his movements are now mechanical and uncertain

. he no longer knows the purpose of a bathroom or bathing, nor how to start washing, showering or bathing

Intervene	. it soon becomes almost impossible for him to recognize, name or indicate a part of his own body, or to raise an arm or leg on request
	. he can no longer connect the soap, the washcloth or the towel with his body or with each other
	. he can no longer wash himself at the lavatory basin; at the most wet his face and hands
	. the pain sensation remains intact
	. see stage I, **bathing** for: expressions of feelings of discomfort, which may indicate giddiness; itching and scratching himself; abnormalities of the skin
Partial take-over	√ put a soaped washcloth in his hand, extend an arm to him and say: "Wash my arm", subsequently: "Now your arm" and simultaneously point to it. Subsequently: "May I wash you now?" and, if the caregiver is a spouse, playfully continue bathing together; if not bathing together, casually take over the washing
	√ to let him wash himself, give him the soaped washcloth and if necessary guide his hand to the part of his body to be washed and make a washing movement
	√ especially with regard to the face and pubic area first let him 'wash' himself and subsequently casually take over the washing action
	√ when possible avoid washing in the standing up position on account of disturbances of the body balance, of coordination and timing of the movements
Total take-over	√ the activities of washing, bathing and showering must now be taken over totally by the caregiver. The patient can no longer adequately perform these actions, which results in self-neglect. Important points with respect to assisting the patient with these activities are:
	- arouse confidence by quietly approaching him with hands open and palms up and guide him to the bathroom while you talk to him, taking him by the hand
	- avoid grabbing, pushing or pulling the patient, do not compel him to join in doing something which he does not understand and resists

Total take-over

- in the bathroom, show him what he has to do by gesturing and addressing him in a friendly way
- adjust the pace of the activity to the patient's physical movements. All passive movements of each part of the body should be unhurried, equable and flowing, in order to prevent an involuntary resistance of joints resulting from increased muscular tension. Moving a part of his body unexpectedly, erratically and too quickly engenders fear. It then seems as though the patient is obstinate and is putting up resistance
√ preferably use a handhold shower head and direct the jet of water first to his feet and gradually allow it to come higher via the side of the body. Prevent the jet of water from touching his face

Attitude

√ realize that washing, bathing and showering no longer have any more point for him. Water is to him something elusive; its form and temperature are always changing. Moreover water is a hindrance to the patient's sight and hearing while showering and thus may cause unstable balance and increasing fear, which can lead to panic
√ realize that continuing to perform even the most simple action gives the patient a certain degree of control over the situation, which can diminish anxiety and resistance
√ think the activity through beforehand and examine the way in which the patient may react and how in such a case the actions can be performed
√ gain his confidence by radiating friendliness, calm and patience, whereby his body moves less rigidly
√ keep calm if the patient is angry; avoid showing uncertainty and fear yourself, causing even more panic in the patient and resistance, while the caregiver also gets tense
√ recognize the difference between manhandling and gently touching the patient

What the patient can do himself

√ act on extremely simple and explicit instructions

√ show what he finds agreeable and disagreeable, spontaneously and on request: laugh, give a kiss, stiffen, or hit out

√ move spontaneously, but often not on request:
  . from lying down to standing to remaining standing to starting to walk
  . from walking to standing still, but usually with difficulty or not at all from standing to sitting to lying down

√ sometimes undress himself on request

√ when invited by his caregiver:
  . put his hand or foot into a hand extended to him
  . get in and out of the bath or shower

√ on request, adapt his posture to a necessary activity to a certain extent and maintain the position for a short period during the washing activity, for instance:
  . hold up his arms and legs
  . keep his legs apart
  . remain standing
  . bend his lower back slightly forward
  . roll over from his back on to his stomach and vice versa

√ indicate the presence, but not the location of pain and discomfort in groans and shrieks

Intervene observe for, and if necessary prevent

√ fear and agitation during showering or bathing:
  . he is no longer aware that he has a back and no longer recognizes a chair as an object to sit on. Having his bottom and surrounding area washed by the caregiver is often experienced as a threat to which he reacts with fear
  . since he is no longer capable of forming an idea of what is going to happen, he is unsure and easily frightened; he has lost all sense of control of the situation and is consequently unable to cooperate and adjust his body to the demands made on it by the caregiver
  . he can no longer stand on one foot without the support of another person and with support only for a short time
  . he easily loses his equilibrium by bending too far forward or too far sideways when sitting

Intervene   √ the patient's fragile skin resulting from:
- poor circulation with stasis and swelling of the lower legs
- atrophy of the epidermis: shiny,thin, dry, yellowish and less resilient skin
- increased fragility of blood vessels with the appearance of blue spots
- excessive formation of wrinkles caused by weight loss or dehydration
- pressure sores related to prolonged sitting and lying down in the same position
- use of certain medicines, which can cause rashes
- repeated shifting over the seat of the chair and sinking back in the chair
- creases in his clothes

Partial take-over   √ when helping him to sit down, see that the chair cannot slip away and that the patient's lower back rests against the back of the chair. Be tactful in the way help is offered. For a specific technique to help the patient to sit down, see the appendix 'Prevention of Falls'

Total take-over   √ prevent bedsores:
- see that there is a cushion in the (wheel)chair which exerts varying pressure on the buttocks and prevents the edge of the seat from cutting into the back of the upper legs
- adjust the footrests of the wheelchair to such a height that the pressure of the body is divided over the patient's seat and the back of the upper legs. In the case of absent or too low footrests, the weight of the legs causes the pressure to increase at the midlevel of the upper legs, and the patient slides forward in the chair. He then has to regularly push himself up on his arms in order to be able to sit comfortably. In this case, the edge of the seat also compresses the bloodvessels and nerves in the upper leg which may lead to painful neuropathy and circulatory disturbance with premature loss of ambulatory ability. If the footrests are too high, the upper legs lose contact with the cushion and the

point of maximum pressure shifts to the nodes of the
buttocks and the seat sacrum, which increases the
chance of bedsores and pain
- regularly check the points of pressure, especially the
  seat, elbows, heels, inside of the knees and ankles
- carefully wash and pat dry a soiled anus and genitals
- see that there is dry, clean underwear and that underwear
  and outerwear are pulled smoothly over the patient's seat
- encourage patients who spend long periods in a chair to
  stand for a moment about four times an hour
- lift the patient instead of pushing him back into the
  chair; a chafing movement damages the skin
- keep the bottom sheet of his bed free of creases and
  crumbs
- when using an extra bottom sheet, place it so that the
  edges do not touch the patient's back, seat and heels
- place the blanket in such a way that the patient retains
  full freedom of movement and an unobstructed view

Attitude   √ realize your responsibility with regard to the prevention
of decubitus (bedsores). Decubitus, bedsores or pressure
sores, is the damage done to the skin and underlying
tissue at places where the bone lies just under the skin.
Decubitus is caused by short-lived major pressure or
long-lasting minor pressure and constant shifting or
chafing and can in principle occur in any place in the
body. In particular chairbound patients have a higher
chance of suffering from decubitus, especially on their
seat and on their elbows, on which they often lean
√ decubitus causes:
. pain
. infection of underlying tissues
. chronic loss of blood and protein
. weakening of the physical and psychosocial resistance
. restricted movement and increased rigidity
. increased dependency
. a more difficult task for the caregiver
. it often heals very slowly and may become chronic

What the patient can do himself

√ bend and stretch the hands and fingers and manipulate objects with some control
√ sometimes polish fingernails (women)
√ wash and dry the hands and apply hand cream
√ on request reach out the right or left hand

Intervene observe for, and prevent

√ cold, stiff, swollen or painful fingers, resulting in a greatly diminished sense of touch
√ sharp protrusions from edge of nails; loose skin of cuticle
√ chapped hands; cuts; skin rash, eczema
√ painful and swollen finger and wrist joints
√ dirty hands and nails

Partial take-over

√ frequent stimulation to perform hand, finger and wrist exercises, also to prevent contracture of the joints
√ accompany him to wash his hands after going to the toilet, meals and other activities

Total take-over

√ clean fingernails on surface and underneath; cut and file nails
√ daily massage of his hands, fingers and wrists. This has various advantages:
- the massage promotes contact
- it has a soothing and relaxing effect on the patient
- it has a stimulating effect on the circulation of the blood, so that the often cold hands become warm again
- it provides the opportunity of inspecting the skin of the fingers for dryness, temperature, smoothness
- it makes it possible to observe changes in movement of the hands and fingers

Attitude

√ realize that continuing to perform hand movements is of great importance for the functioning of the patient. His hands are his principal link with the world
√ realize that the sense of touch is experienced above all through the fingers. Fingers which can touch and feel are extremely important for the maintenance of contact with the outside world and for maintaining functions which have not yet been lost

What the patient can do himself	√ perform simple, crude hand and finger movements of thumb and fingers together √ wash and dry his hands
Intervene	√ his fingers sometimes have an inclination towards curling up in the palm of the hand
Total take-over	√ massage of hands, fingers and wrists: - put your hand on the back of the patient's hand and make rubbing movements, wait a moment before taking hold of his hand - subsequently take his hand with the fingers stretched between your own two hands. Avoid stimulating the palm of his hand; this causes a grasping reflex - using both hands, massage the back of the patient's hands and his fingers with your fingers for at least five minutes; rub, vibrate, stroke, knead and gently straighten out the fingers. Also massage the back of the wrist and each finger and the thumb separately

What the
patient can
do himself

√ put his foot in another person's hand reached out
    to him
√ sometimes distinguish between the right and left shoe
√ indicate pain

Intervene
observe for,
and if neces-
sary prevent

√ difficulties or discomfort with walking resulting from:
  . holes in shoes, stockings, panty hose or socks
  . doubled up lining sole of shoe
  . too large or too small shoes
  . cold feet
  . chilblains
  . long toenails
  . ingrown toenails
  . brittle nails
  . corns
  . calluses under the ball of the foot or edge of the heel
  . blisters
  . athletes foot
  . eczema
  . cuts between the toes
  . painful, swollen joints (i.e., from gout)
  . swollen ankles (edema)
  . varicose veins

Total
take-over

√ wash his feet daily and dry them well, especially
  between the toes to prevent skin irritation and itching
√ let him wear shoes instead of slippers
√ put on clean socks, stockings or panty hose every day
√ check the inside of his shoes for any unevenness
√ cut toenails short and straight across; round off corners
√ if necessary see a podiatrist in the case of malformations
√ daily massage of feet and ankles:
  - massage promotes contact
  - it has a soothing and relaxing effect on the patient

**What the
patient can
do himself**
√ put his foot into another person's hand reached out
to him
√ express pain if this occurs by putting pressure on the
foot or toenails

Intervene
√ the patient can no longer stand on one foot
√ the patient can no longer stand on his toes

**Total
take-over**
√ daily massage of his feet and ankles. See also
Stage III A, **hand care**
√ the technique of foot massage:
1 place a hand on the patient's foot and make a rubbing
movement, wait a moment before taking hold of his
foot
2 take his foot in both hands. Holding the foot
reasonably firmly prevents a ticklish feeling
3 massage the foot with both hands for at least five
minutes; rub, vibrate, stroke and knead with your
fingers over his foot and ankles

Attitude
√ realize that the patient is still able to walk
independently for several years, provided he has no
complicating conditions of his legs and feet
√ realize that with good foot care and well fitting shoes,
ambulation is maintained
√ realize that the patient often has an urge to walk

What the
patient can
do himself

during stage IIIA he can:

√ on request:
. point to his mouth and teeth
. open and shut his mouth
. keep his mouth open for a short time and put out his
   tongue
. breathe deeply in and out
. bite
. chew
. swallow
. spit out
. blow
. wipe his mouth

√ recognize his mirror image

√ with some control of the manipulatory finger
  movements, use the toothbrush, clean his teeth and
  rinse the brush

√ pick up the water glass, take a sip of water, rinse his
  mouth and spit the water out again

√ put his dentures in his mouth and take them out

Encourage
patient to

√ induce action by means of inviting gestures,
  indication and presentation of requisites, and explicit
  prompting:
. " take hold of – this brush"
. " clean/brush – there too"
. " pick up that glass – drink – do not swallow – spit
   out"
. " put that brush down – there"
. " take hold of – this cloth – wipe off – your mouth"
. " may I have your dentures – that one too"
. "take hold of – dentures – put into your mouth" (pass
   upper and lower dentures separately)

√ it sometimes helps if the caregiver brushes his own
  teeth and invites the patient to perform the same
  activity on himself

√ at the dentist the patient can open his mouth and keep
  it open for a very short time only

√ when taking medicine prompt him: "pick this up, put it in your mouth, chew or swallow, take this glass, drink". When a patient refuses to take medication, it sometimes helps if the caregiver takes his own medication or a placebo at the same time

Intervene
observe for, and if neces-sary prevent

√ failure to wear the dentures regularly leads to getting out of the habit and finally to rejection of the dentures (see stage II)

√ tooth decay: Fairly soon within the course of this stage the patient becomes unable to cooperate with the dentist because he no longer understands the dentist's requests and indications. He can only maintain a particular pose or action for a short time. An agitated patient with an acute dental problem requires sedation

Partial take-over

√ put out all necessary requisites
√ put toothpaste on the brush
√ clean the brush after use
√ check whether the dentures are firmly in his mouth
√ prevent drying out of the mucus membrane of the mouth and see that his breath is fresh (see stage I)

Total take-over

√ the care of the dentures (see stage II)
√ good oral hygiene:
  - let him clean his teeth and rinse his mouth well, preferably with a mouthwash, three times a day, or
  - clean his dentures and let him rinse his mouth, preferably with a mouthwash, three times a day
  - keep his lips greased to prevent drying out and the formation of cracks in his lips
  - clean the corners of the mouth
  - let him drink at least 3 pints of fluid per day

Attitude

√ realize that bad breath is an impediment to touching and kissing the patient
√ realize that oral and dental problems can be a cause of slow eating or refusal of food

What the patient can do himself

√ after many repeated requests, accompanied by gestures: open and shut his mouth; stick his tongue out for a short time; chew; spit out

√ make rubbing movements over his teeth with the toothbrush

√ take a sip of water into his mouth and swallow it

√ take his dentures out of his mouth

√ often still recognize his mirror image

Encourage

√ hand the toothbrush with toothpaste on it, point to his mouth and say:" open your mouth – there – clean your teeth"

√ standing next to him, clean your own teeth and encourage him to imitate you

√ if he cannot do this, take the cleaning activity over from him, saying: "Shall we try it together?"

√ some patients reflexively open their mouth when an object approaches it. This reflex can be utilized in inducing opening of the mouth by slowly and visibly approaching his mouth with a toothbrush (or a spoon with the necessary medication)

Intervene observe for, and if necessary prevent

√ looking into his mouth, cleaning his teeth or swallowing medicine often present problems because the patient no longer understands the request or because of oral apraxia, i.e., no longer knowing how to perform movements with the mouth. Toothpaste, mouthwash, medicines etc. are judged by their taste (pleasant or unpleasant) and accordingly swallowed or spat out

√ choking; he is:

. sometimes unable to spit out mouthwash or chewing gum

. sometimes unable to completely suck a candy

. unable to swallow medicines whole which are in the form of capsules or coated tablets

√ see for prevention of choking and what to do in the event of choking stage IV, **eating and drinking**

**Total
take-over**

√ the final cleaning of his teeth

√ clean his dentures three times a day and regularly inspect them for damage. Badly fitting dentures are painful

√ put his dentures into his mouth. Give breath refresher (such as mint tea)

What the patient can do himself	√ recognize his own mirror image √ wash and dry his face, neck and ears on request √ apply soap, cream, lipstick on request √ on request, and if the item is visible and within reach: pick up comb, hairbrush, a piece of soap and shaver (he is often no longer able to name them) √ comb his hair √ shave himself in the way he is used to; apply shaving cream or use the electric shaver √ blow his nose in a tissue

Remind and encourage patient to	√ by explicit prompting, to:
	  . "pick up that washcloth, rub your face, rub your neck"
	  . "take that towel, dry your face"
	  . "put that shaving cream on your cheek, pick up that shaver, there, now shave"

Intervene observe for, and if necessary prevent	√ frequent scratching of his head; look for possible causes, such as too dry skin or head lice √ signs of dizziness during and after bending his head back for hair washing. The latter should be done in the sitting position √ eczema; beside his nostrils, in the auditory canal and behind his ears in particular √ bloodshot and inflamed eyes from frequent rubbing √ dry chapped lips √ blocked sebaceous glands √ avoid unnecessary touching of his head as this frightens him Advice: let the facial care actions take place seated in front of a mirror so that he can see what is happening. Promote contact by sitting opposite the patient, at eye level, when giving facial care.

Total take-over

√ accompany patient to the barber or hairdresser
√ comb the hair into shape – trim beard or mustache
√ apply cream or lotion
√ clean the facial skin in the evening and apply a rich cream
√ keep the lips greased, during the day and at night
√ care for ears, eyes and nose, such as cleaning, applying ointment
√ wash and dry his neck and area behind his ears
√ remove long hairs; from chin and upper lip for women; from ears and nose for men
√ if necessary shave off incompletely removed beard. If he frequently cuts himself, take over the shaving completely
√ consult the doctor in the event of persistent abnormalities of the skin, ears, eyes and nose (such as eczema, impacted ear wax, conjunctivitis, running nose)

Attitude

√ continue visiting the barber or hairdresser as long as possible

What the patient can do himself

√ often still recognize his mirror image
√ comb his hair
√ blow his nose himself

Intervene observe for, and if necessary prevent

√ the patient being frightened when his head is touched as with:
  . getting water on his head when bathing
  . washing and combing his hair
  . shaving, especially the upper lip
  . cleaning or putting drops in his eyes, ears or nose
√ he no longer recognizes the sound of the electric shaver as such and therefore often makes turning and searching movements with his head, with the danger of damaging the skin

Total take-over

√ carry out the necessary actions on his head in front of the mirror so that he can see what is happening to him
√ carry out the shaving actions seated and on his eye level
√ show him the electric shaver, plug in, put it into his hand and guide his hand to his face, subsequently casually take over the shaving action
√ do not take hold of him during shaving, only touch him by means of the appliance and if necessary use the other hand to stretch the skin
√ after shaving in front of the mirror let him feel his facial skin with his own hand and give him a compliment

What the patient can do himself

√ on seeing a garment indicate whether or not he wants to put it on

√ indicate discomfort caused by ill fitting clothes

√ move from lying down to sitting to standing to remaining standing to walking and vice versa

√ sit down when requested

√ dress himself independently if he is given the clothes in the correct order; put on a garment which does not change form considerably such as an overcoat, jacket or blazer

√ decide whether he first wants to put his right arm or leg, or his left arm or leg into the sleeve or trouser leg

√ recognize his own mirror image

√ while seated: put on shoes and sometimes socks, but often not stockings or panty hose

√ if garments such as undershorts, trousers, skirt, sweater or nightdress are presented to him spread out, he can:
  . pick them up or take hold of them
  . put his head, hands or feet through the appropriate openings
  . pull the garment on as far as and over the joint and pull it further up or down

√ if the initial impetus is given by holding the sleeve opening of a blouse, shirt or dress in front of the appropriate hand, he can:
  . put his hand in it
  . guide his hand further; find the other sleeve himself
  . pull the garment on as far as and over the joint and pull it further up or down

√ do the garment up by means of a large button and a large buttonhole

Remind and encourage patient to
if necessary explain
step by step

√ first direct his attention to the garment to be put on and then to his own hand. Say: "put your arm in this sleeve"

√ undress before going to bed

√ perform each action step by step and in the right order, indicating each subject of the action explicitly:
. "undo this shoelace"
. "take off, that shoe"
. "put it down, there, that shoe"

√ the patient often no longer knows the order in which the garments successively have to be put on, and he is continually distracted by details or goes on repeating the component actions over and again. Thus he may do up the shoelace again he has just undone or hold the shoe in his hand and keep on feeling it, or he finds fluff on his trouser legs and makes lengthy brushing movements with his hand and stops going on with dressing, etc.

Intervene
observe for

√ possible causes of an inability to dress oneself:
. garments are less and less recognized as belonging on particular parts of the body
. he may no longer know that the bedroom or bathroom are the proper places to get dressed
. he may no longer have any idea of being visible to other people during dressing and undressing
. he only understands extremely simple explicit indications and requests which have an immediate bearing on the situation. The goal of the action, that is: where do I have to go, and the plan of action, that is: how do I get there, are both lost. The patient gets stuck in the component action, does not know how to go on and thus keeps on repeating the component action. He gets nowhere on his own. Prompting by the caregiver for each successive step of the activity is needed in order to achieve the desired result

Partial take-over

√ the dressing actions should be carried out sitting down; performing two different movements simultaneously causes confusion and often one of the movements goes awry, for instance loss of balance when raising his leg and stepping into the trouser leg at the same time

√ spread out the garments in front of the patient one by one and in the right order. Supervise and guide the subsequent actions to be performed by the patient. Smooth out the clothes and do up the fastening

√ sitting on the same eye level when helping the patient to get dressed promotes contact

√ let him get dressed sitting in front of the mirror with his glasses on if necessary, so that he can see what is happening

Total take-over

√ see that the patient puts on:
- her bra
- her panties
- avoids wearing knee socks with tight elastic borders because of pressure on the calves, causing impaired circulation
- her preferred jewelry

√ keep as far as possible to his or her familiar way of dressing

√ find the right balance between letting him do what he is still able to do and offering help. Allow him to be as independent as possible, without leaving him to his own devices

√ during and after dressing check for:
  . too tightly fitting clothes, causing laceration or chafing
  . lacerations from hook and eye fastenings
  . straighten out a wrinkled bottom edge of the garment on which the patient is sitting. This also helps to prevent decubitus

√ after undressing inspect the skin for damage

Attitude √ help the patient to feel as independent as possible by taking hold of him as little as possible during dressing
√ being undressed by another person can be a frightening event, since it means to the patient: 'taking something away from him'. Accompany him quietly to the place where he usually dresses. Let him sit down and, while stroking his back, say: "May I have your sweater?" and simultaneously point to it (do not grab it)
√ always help the patient in a friendly, calm manner; do not show impatience or irritation, because that confuses him and makes him feel inadequate

What the patient can do himself

√ indicate pleasant or unpleasant situations
√ often still recognize his own mirror image
√ experience pain and express it by groaning or shrieking
√ move spontaneously and sometimes on command:
  . from lying down to sitting to standing, remain standing and starting to walk
  . from walking to standing still, but with difficulty from standing to sitting to lying
√ sometimes undress himself on command
√ after the caregiver has put his hand or foot through the appropriate opening of the vest or undershorts, trousers or skirt to just over the first joint, he can pull the garment further up or down

Intervene observe for, and if necessary prevent

√ inability to stand on one foot without support, such as standing alone to step into a trouser leg
√ resisting the caregiver in undressing him, though he can still do it himself
√ rough opening or overstretching of the joints when dressing
√ lacerating, constricting or chafing clothing
√ at the end of this stage he can no longer automatically follow the dressing movements. The caregiver has to steer and if necessary support the joints while guiding the garment over them

Total take-over

√ when assisting the patient, move each part of the body slowly and smoothly, in order to prevent sudden stiffening of the joints due to the occurrence of heightened muscular tension. Moving a part of the body unexpectedly, erratically and too quickly causes pain and sometimes panic. It may seem as though the patient is actively resisting and refusing to cooperate. In fact the joints become locked due to sudden reflexive muscular tension. Do not force the arm or leg into stretching or bending, but relax the tension by massaging the arm or leg muscles and simultaneously slowly and evenly stretching or bending the extremity

Attitude   √ realize that in order to cooperate with the care giver the
patient needs to have insight into what the caregiver
wants from him. This insight is entirely lacking in the
patient. He is not able to cooperate and cannot be
blamed for it

What the patient can do himself

√ in words:
  . ask for food and drink when hungry or thirsty
  . refuse food and drink
  . indicate pain in the mouth or stomach
  . make it clear that he must go to the toilet
  . indicate whether food and drink are too hot or too cold
  . say familiar prayers on appropriate occasions, such as saying grace before and after meals

√ sitting at the table, pick up something which is straight in front of him at arm's-length, bring it towards him and put it on his plate

√ butter a piece of toast

√ sometimes eat with a knife and fork and cut soft food

√ spear, push and scoop with the fork

√ push and scoop with the spoon

√ put a spoon with semi-liquid food into his mouth without spilling

√ drink from a cup, glass or mug without spilling

√ suck up a drink with a straw

√ put food in his mouth with his fingers

√ lick up food with his tongue

√ chew coarse bread, meat, raw vegetables and fruit

√ wipe his mouth on his table napkin on request

√ fetch food from the cupboard or refrigerator if hungry or thirsty

Remind and encourage patient to

√ go to the toilet before the meal

√ put on and keep on his glasses, so that he can see what is on his plate, the tableware and his table-companions

√ continue his meal or eat more slowly and chew well by prompting: "take – this slice of bread" "take – that knife there – take the butter there – spread it" "take – that fork there" "take that glass – drink" "take hold of – this cloth – wipe your mouth"

Intervene
observe for,
and if neces-
sary prevent

√ leaving the table constantly: satisfying his hunger is no
longer bound up with the three daily meals. He leaves
the table if he is uncomfortable, has no appetite, does
not like the food, does not receive enough attention or
is distracted

√ cutlery and crockery which he has put in front of him
is not put back again

√ a shifting plate presents a major obstacle for him

√ he cannot choose, because he cannot distinguish the
items of food from one another. Only through the taste
is he able to decide what he likes or does not like

√ some patients may eat ravenously, resulting in air being
swallowed, leading to dilation of the stomach and loss
of appetite, causing him to stop eating before he has
had enough food. It may result in loss of weight. In
such cases distracting the patient may reduce the pace
of eating

√ sometimes food is refused for fear of being poisoned,
possibly because the sense of taste has become
disturbed

√ taking food off someone else's plate because he feels
hungry, sees food and cannot distinguish between mine
and thine any more

**Partial
take-over**

√ indicate the order of the dishes for the meal to
the patient. Put the dishes in front of him one by one
with the appropriate cutlery

√ if necessary, divide the food into small pieces, but do
not cut it up fine or mix it all up together

√ serve him seasoning, such as sugar, salt, ketchup

√ serve soup in a soup bowl or cup and fill it half full.
Plastic crockery and cutlery is too light-weight and
should be avoided

√ remove bones and sinews from meat; bones from fish;
stones from fruit

**Total
take-over**

√ Three times a day at set times, eat with the patient
at a properly laid table. Meals help structurize the day's
schedule

√ see that there is comfortable seating: a heavier chair
with long armrests and soft stuffing in the seat. A
slightly backward leaning seat with stiff upholstery
prevents sliding forward. If the chair is adjusted to the
posture of the patient, his back, bottom and the whole
of his upper leg are supported while he is sitting and
the soles of his feet are in contact with the floor. The
height of the dining table is important in connection
with stretching his trunk; there must be no
impediments to the region of the stomach nor to
respiration during the meal

√ direct restlessness at table into good channels:
before the meal:
. go to the toilet
. wash the hands
. comb the hair in front of the mirror and compliment
  the patient on his or her appearance
during the meal, provide a friendly ambiance:
. soft background music
. laughing together
after the meal:
. sitting still for 15 minutes is necessary to prevent
  giddiness and falling if the patient stands up too soon

√ eat with the patient if he is suffering from a delusion of
being poisoned. Taking it in turns, demonstratively eat
a mouthful of the same portion. Or, if that does not
have any effect, remove the food and distract him. The
delusion often disappears if he is distracted and the
meal can then be continued

Attitude   √ realize that eating a meal together at the laid table is a
                  social happening. If the patient is made to eat from a
                  small table attached to the wheelchair and is then
                  helped with certain actions, one is reminded of a big
                  child in the highchair. For the patient it can represent
                  estrangement, restriction of freedom, isolation,
                  powerlessness, deprivation of action and no longer
                  being accepted as a table companion. As long as the
                  patient is able to walk (up to the middle of stage IV),
                  being confined to a wheelchair means diminution of
                  his world, dependence and premature loss of
                  ambulation

What the patient can do himself	√ walk to the dining table by himself √ leave the table by himself √ ineffectively change seats; get up and immediately sit down again and wiggle to and fro √ when sitting at the table, reach out for something at arm's-length, take hold of it and bring it towards him √ scoop up food with spoon and fork √ spear larger pieces with his fork √ drink from a cup, glass or mug without spilling √ chew small portions slowly √ suck up a drink with a straw √ put food in his mouth with his fingers √ lick up food with his tongue √ chew coarse bread, meat, raw vegetable or fruit provided the pieces are small and his teeth are in good condition √ indicate refusal of food and drink by means of gestures and keeping his mouth tightly shut
Remind and encourage patient to	√ sit down at the table √ start eating √ continue eating or eat slower √ drink √ wipe his mouth
Intervene observe for, and if necessary prevent	√ the patient losing weight because he is unable to fetch food or beverage for himself if he is hungry or thirsty and no longer recognizes the laid table as a place to eat √ sometimes he is unable to distinguish between what is edible and what is inedible √ a pained expression on his face, tightly pursed lips as when tasting something bitter or acid. This may indicate a painful tooth or an oral infection. The only way in which the patient can refuse food is to push it away, knock it out of the caregiver's hands or start shrieking. If the patient's mouth is not adequately inspected an important reason for his not wanting to eat may be ignored

Intervene   √ *dehydration:* because of inadequate fluid intake or excessive fluid loss. He looks ill, feels cold and is apathetic. Dehydration can be recognized by:
. very dry and easily tenting rimpled skin, sometimes with a bluish tint
. sunken eyes, with a dim gaze
. a faint rapid pulse
. diminished or ceased production of urine
. in serious cases, delirium, seizures and coma can occur, as well as respiratory problems. Dehydration is a medical emergency

√ a rigid and flexed or overextended neck may seriously impair the patient's ability to swallow. Occasionally, neuroleptics may aggravate this problem (dystonia of the neck)

Partial take-over   √ maintain routine of eating at the table three meals a day at the same times in stead of giving the patient his meal at the place he happens to be sitting and at the moment he indicates to be hungry. Regularity in the place, the time and the duration of the meal is of importance for a good digestion and maintenance of eating habits

√ put the sandwich cut into small pieces in front of him with or without a fork

√ cut potatoes, vegetable and meat into small pieces, but do not mince or puree it or mix it all up together

√ serve soup, yoghurt, custard in a mug with two handles to avoid spilling

√ give the patient three pints of liquid a day. Older people often fail to drink enough because the sensation of thirst diminishes, which can lead to confusion, drowsiness, staggering, his knees giving way, fainting, a dry mouth and difficulty in swallowing. Major loss of fluid can only be replenished in the hospital by intravenous administration. If the treatment of dehydration is left too late or is inadequate, innumerable complications occur. With disturbances of the balance of fluid disturbances of the balance of salt also occur. Dehydration is a life threatening condition which calls for emergency admittance to hospital

Total take-over

√ if the patient eats poorly or will not eat at all, look for possible causes, such as:
  . physical problems, such as fever, pain
  . distracting surroundings
  . dislike of particular food
  . medicines which make it difficult to swallow (such as neuroleptics)
  . not chewing properly and eating ravenously

√ do not put an apron on the patient during the meal. To protect his clothes from getting messy, push the armrests of the chair right against the table and fasten a large table napkin round his neck, with the stiffly starched edge of the napkin folded outwards and resting on his knees

√ provide solid cutlery with thicker and longer handles

√ use a nonslip mat to prevent the plate and mug from sliding away

√ see that there is enough to drink; the patient will not ask for it

√ use suitable drinking vessels

√ check on side effects of medicines (in particular diuretics, sedatives or neuroleptics)

√ let him drink a certain amount of fluid such as mineral water at set times

√ make a 24-hour fluid balance list. Note carefully how much he drinks and how much urine he passes. If the intake of fluid is about four pints, then the release of urine should be about 2 1/2 pints per 24 hours. If the patient is incontinent, the amount of urine can be roughly determined by weighing the wet material

√ regular check on the body weight

√ problems with drinking causing insufficient fluid intake and a resulting drop in the urine production may herald dehydration. Consultation with a physician or nurse is called for

√ make sure that he wears a clean incontinence system before he starts eating

Attitude   √ realize that trying to suppress the urge to move by the use of a restraint band has a contrary effect. The patient becomes more restless and agitated, offers resistance, does not eat or does not finish his meal, and afterwards goes looking for something to eat because he is still hungry

√ realize that the patient cannot indicate that he is thirsty. A sudden change in the level of consciousness, with increased drowsiness and inactivity, is usually the first symptom of dehydration. The chance of dehydration is great when warm humid weather conditions prevail. Inflammatory conditions, fever, diarrhea, vomiting, diabetes, use of diuretics, tranquillizers or neuroleptics are also potential causes of dehydration because there is an increased need for, an insufficient intake of, or an excess loss of fluid from the body

What the patient can do himself

√ by means of word or gesture:
  . make it clear that he must go to the toilet
  . indicate discomfort in the pubic area or anus
√ in his own home go to the toilet on becoming aware of the urge and feelings of discomfort in the bladder or stomach
√ recognize the toilet as the appropriate place to urinate and defecate
√ zip the fly open and urinate standing up
√ before and after going to the toilet pull clothes up or down; sometimes zip up the fly
√ sit on and stand up from the toilet bowl
√ clean the anus with toilet paper
√ throw the used paper in the toilet bowl
√ flush the toilet
√ wash and dry his hands

Remind and encourage patient to

√ as long as he still understands simple commands, instruct him to perform in succession:
√ while seated, wipe the anus after the bowel movement with toilet paper
√ subsequently throw the used paper in the toilet bowl
√ subsequently pull up his undershorts
√ subsequently pull up and zip up his trousers or pull her skirt down
√ subsequently flush the toilet
√ subsequently wash his hands

Intervene observe for, and if necessary prevent

√ potentially redressable causes of incontinence, such as:
- being unable to get to the toilet in time because of physical reasons
- when feeling the urge, go to the toilet, but having arrived there no longer know what to do
- when feeling the urge, search for the toilet, but unable to find the toilet door
- being frightened of sitting down on the toilet seat, because, possibly, the toilet bowl represents a hole with water and something you can sag into

Intervene   - being frightened of going to the toilet because of pain
                when urinating and/or defecating
              √ signs indicating an urge to urinate or defecate, such as:
                becoming restless; rubbing his arms and legs; touching
                the pubic area or the anus, raising the skirt or pulling it
                tightly down over the knees, opening the fly,
                continually pressing the knees together
              √ fecal impaction: if a constipated patient can suddenly
                no longer hold his feces and the latter is diarrhea-like, it
                can be that hard excrement has accumulated in the
                rectum and partially blocks the intestine. Soft
                excrement collects above this. Through the effect of
                bacteria the hard, dried-in excrement can partially
                soften again. At intervals soft feces escape via the
                slackened, enlarged, often open sphincter. The patient
                then has what is called 'paradoxical diarrhea'. The
                greatest mistake which can then be made is to give the
                patient an antidiarrheal, because in this case the
                constipation is the cause of the diarrhea. Laxatives are
                equally harmful in such a situation. With paradoxical
                diarrhea the feces are sometimes thicker and are not
                then completely absorbed by clothing or bedding, as
                with diarrea proper. Nausea and vomiting, abdominal
                distension, hypotension and an acute confusional state
                may occur with this condition. Paradoxical diarrhea
                and fecal impaction predominate in chairbound or
                bedbound patients, in particular when these patients
                receive psychotropic medication, laxatives or antacids.
                It constitutes a medical emergency and requires
                immediate clinical evaluation. Constipation and fecal
                impaction can often be prevented by adequate fluid
                intake and food which contains sufficient amounts of
                vegetable fiber

Partial take-over

√ leave the toilet door open and switch on the light

√ give him privacy during the act of urination and defecation

√ after the evacuation of the bowel, pass the toilet paper and give instructions for wiping himself, throwing used paper in the toilet bowl and flushing the toilet when he fails to do so

√ adjust his clothing prior to, and after going to the toilet

√ accompany him to the lavatory basin, turn the faucet on and off and give him soap and towel

√ do not let him sit on the toilet for more than ten minutes, because :
  - it can be painful and cause skin irritation through the pressure of the toilet seat
  - it can arouse cramp in his legs
  - it can worsen discomfort from hemorrhoids
  - it can lead to a fall through the trousers dropping round the knees or ankles
  - it may reinforce feelings of fear
  - it can lead to him dirtying himself on account of touching himself as a result of feelings of discomfort

√ check whether he has had a bowel movement and whether this was of a normal consistency. Hard feces may cause disorders in the anal region, such as tears or hemorrhoids, which can in turn lead to hemorrhage. Retarded evacuation of the rectum leads to retarded evacuation of the stomach and may cause pyrosis, nausea and a bloated feeling which decrease the appetite

Total
take-over

√ accompany him to the toilet regularly, at set times
√ if he refuses to sit on the toilet bowl, try a commode, preferably one with a high back and long armrests
√ make use of a toilet hightener, adjusted to his posture, with a hollow at the front
√ to make turning round easier for the patient use can be made of a turntable with a diameter of approximately 40 cm (16 inches) as an aid to shifting position, with the following stipulations: the turntable must not move while the patient is getting onto it; the patient should be supported while getting onto it; his back should be slowly and gradually turned to the toilet bowl by means of the movement of the turntable
√ have the urine checked periodically to exclude urinary tract infection as a cause of urine incontinence
√ when he can no longer wipe himself, clean the anus by stroking with soft toilet paper or a damp washcloth, from the anus in the direction of the lower back. In women, cystitis can be caused by bacteria from the feces finding their way into the ureter and bladder
√ make a daily note of bowel movements
√ in the event of incontinence at night only:
  - let him drink three pints of liquid per day, but
  - do not give him any tea, coffee or diuretics in the evening
  - let him sit with his legs raised several times during the day to prevent pooling in the legs of fluid, which has to be expelled at night. It may decrease the urge to urinate at night
  - do not give him anything more to drink from two hours before going to bed
  - let him go to the toilet before going to bed
  - one accompanied visit to the toilet during the night may decrease restlessness
  - the administration of diuretics as prescribed by the physician
  - in the event of persisting problems with urination, such as too little, too often, painful or difficult urination, consult the physician

Attitude

√ give him as much privacy as possible while he relieves himself

√ do not reproach him if he is incontinent or breaks wind, since he is no longer aware of it himself

√ let him perform all actions which he can still carry out himself.

√ be aware that prolonged constipation, in particular when associated with confusion and agitation, may constitute a medical emergency

What the patient can do himself

√ follow frequently repeated, extremely simple instructions
√ indicate unpleasant sensations
√ indicate the urge to urinate or defecate, by putting his hand on the pubic area and/or lower his trousers wherever he happens to be or open the fly and relieve himself
√ change spontaneously, and sometimes on repeated request:
. from lying down to sitting to standing to remaining standing and starting to walk
. from walking to standing still, with difficulty from standing to sitting to lying
. in the lying down position, roll over from his stomach to his back and vice versa
√ with the guidance of the caregiver:
. pull down and put pull up his trousers with two hands
. turn round, sit down and stand up from the toilet bowl
. urinate standing up
√ by means of groans or shrieks express feelings of discomfort, such as pain, itching, dizziness, cramp in the legs or pain in the rectum, sitting uncomfortably and fear of falling when sitting
√ wash his hands with liquid soap put on his hands and dry his hands with a towel

Remind and encourage patient to

√ perform the necessary actions sequentially by first directing his attention to the garment, and then to his hands and subsequently to his seat and upper legs:
. pull the pants down or open the zipper, pull the skirt up
. turn with his seat towards the toilet bowl and stand so that the calves or hollow of the knees touch the bowl
. while holding up his clothes, bend his body slightly forward and let his seat protrude backwards. Then say: "sit down"
. move the upper legs slightly apart to prevent urinating over the edge of the bowl
. keep his feet flat on the floor

Intervene
observe for,
and if neces-
sary prevent

√ the patient no longer knows what a toilet bowl is for, nor why or how to use it. The discharge of urine and feces is now also totally uncontrolled and involuntary. He no longer realizes that the discharge of urine and feces is about to take place. The urge often takes the patient by surprise and he has to answer nature's call immediately. He can no longer decide to relieve himself, it just happens. That is why a discharge takes place somewhere where it does not belong. He no longer has any idea that this is socially unacceptable and can therefore no longer offer his excuses for what has happened. He does however experience discomfort

√ he no longer knows that he must turn round in order to sit down

√ in the event of a great deal of resistance and anxiety about sitting down on the toilet, do not force him but let him relieve himself in the incontinence system

√ the cellulose of the incontinence system must have adequate power of absorption, so that the urine is quickly absorbed and the skin remains dry. The system must not slip down when the patient walks. An average elderly adult produces about two quarts of urine per day. The bladder can hold a maximum amount of approximately one pint. For men, use is sometimes also made of a condom urinal, which is fitted round the penis to lead the urine into a bag attached to the upper leg

√ an indwelling catheter: this is a soft rubber tube inserted into the bladder and which remains there for the regular discharge of urine;

. possible complications of the indwelling catheter are:
   - inflammation of and bulges (diverticula) in the wall of the urethra
   - inflammation and decubitus of, and stones in the bladder
   - blockage of the lumen of the catheter, resulting in damming up of urine in the bladder and kidneys, with resultant infection of these organs
   - leakage along the catheter, resulting in urine being squeezed alongside the catheter

Intervene   - damage to the ureter and bladder on account of the patient pulling on the catheter, so that it has to be renewed frequently
- irritation of the skin and sometimes decubitus on account of sitting on the catheter

Partial take-over   √ prevent soiling of himself and his surroundings from feces by:
- maintaining regular visits to the toilet as long as possible
- noting the time at which urination and bowel movement usually take place and accompanying him to the toilet every day at that time
- seeing that there is supervision and help before, during and after the evacuation
- making a daily note of the estimated amount, consistency and color of the feces
- regularly inspecting the area round the rectum for irritation, hemorrhoids and threadworms; providing good skin care. With feelings of discomfort from constipation, itching or pain the patient keeps on touching the rectum, resulting in soiling himself and his surroundings
- regularly having his hands washed and nails inspected

Total take-over   √ incontinence and the accompanying care:
- let him drink three pints of liquid per day and make a note of the amount given
- prevent dehydration, with the resultant confusion and drowsiness. In dry or very warm surroundings, excess loss of fluid through the skin can sharply increase
- wash all sweat and urine off the skin; especially in the groins, abdominal fold, genitals, anal cleft, buttocks, to prevent skin irritation
- rinse well after use of soap to prevent irritation of the skin
- dry by dabbing; rubbing can cause irritation

**Total-
take-over**

- gently rub lotion into the skin to prevent dehydration. The use of talcum powder on damp or moistened skin causes the powder to granulate, which can irritate the skin
- change the incontinence system several times a day in order to:
  . prevent ascending infections of the urinary passages, caused by lying or sitting in urine or feces for any length of time
  . prevent discomfort in the patient
  . prevent skin infection and decubitus of the sacral area and buttocks
- prevent skin infection by cleaning the toilet seat before and after use of the toilet, and by always washing the patient's and one's own hands after toileting

√ change the incontinence system in the toilet or bathroom, because:
- in a room with proper facilities at hand the patient can be cared for efficiently and with respect
- the soiled incontinence system can be properly disposed of at the same time. The smell of urine and feces clings to clothes, curtains and upholstery and is difficult to get rid of.

CHAPTER 5

STAGE IV

TOTAL TAKE-OVER

This stage of the disease is characterized by a gradual, and eventually total cessation of all speech, all mobility and all self-awareness. At the onset of this stage the patient not only is no longer able to react adequately to the urge to urinate or defecate; he is now also totally oblivious to the urge itself. For about two years he has not been able to wash himself unassisted. For between two and three years he has needed help with dressing. For six years someone else has managed his financial affairs for him and more than ten years have passed since the earliest symptoms of the disease made their appearance.

The mechanisms of the brain have now deteriorated to such an extent that the patient only has a few short standard sentences or acquired courtesy phrases at his disposal, such as: "Very well, thank you," or "I beg your pardon". His vocabulary diminishes subsequently to a single word which serves to express everything. Finally he may also lose that one word and is then only able to emit sounds, such as grunts, moans or shrieks. If he gets excited, he can sometimes suddenly utter certain explosive sounds in rapid succession, reminiscent of a baby's babbling.

During the first two to three years of this stage, he can still walk independently. He often has an urge to move incessantly, almost the only form of activity left to him. Thus he walks to and fro in the house or through the corridors of the nursing home, room in, room out, taking small steps, putting his forefoot or his whole foot on the floor simultaneously, leaning slightly forward, with his arms held stiffly bent beside his body or held out in front of him, like someone who is groping in the dark. When he comes across an obstacle, or when suddenly confronted with a darker or lighter area, he hesitates, turns round with small steps and walks back. He can sometimes walk like this for hours, alone, or hand in hand with a fellow inmate of the nursing home. Sometimes he drags various objects along with him, such as empty boxes, remains of food, a pillow or personal belongings. He rummages through drawers and bedside cupboards, takes out the contents and puts them down somewhere else. He fumbles for door knobs as if to find a way out. If a caregiver takes the precaution of putting him in a special chair with a board in front to prevent him from falling, he starts to shriek or bang on the the board until he is released. Aimless movement is virtually the only action left to him, in which he can experience himself to any extent. He still reacts when spoken to and smiles at visitors. His facial movements also decrease considerably and he often displays a blank stare. Sometimes a faint smile may appear. Grimacing, such as when in pain or for no obvious reason, is the only facial expression left in the end. He now often keeps his mouth open, unable to close it. Periodic chewing or licking movements sometimes occur.

Initially, he can still use a spoon to bring the food from the plate in front of him into his mouth. But it gradually goes ever more slowly and messily. Eventually, the action becomes impossible, when the connection between spoon and food can no longer be made. Sometimes he can then still eat with his hands, but usually the caregiver has to feed him. He can no longer distinguish between food and substances which are not intended for consumption, and may put everything into his mouth indiscriminately, including, sometimes, his own feces. His eyes can no longer converge on an object. Focussing and depth vision are seriously impaired and he has to grope for objects in front of him.

Then comes the second phase of the last stage. The mechanism of the brain which subserves locomotion is now dysfunctional to such a degree, that independent walking becomes impossible. The balance reflexes are seriously impaired, and are only sufficient to keep the stationary body upright. Only when supported under both arms is the patient able to make stepping and scissoring movements like those of a newborn baby. The patient is now permanently chairbound. His body is now rigid, and it stiffens even more when suddenly taken hold of. Gentle stroking of his limbs by the caregiver can to some extent alleviate the rigidity. Gradually, the balance reflexes become inadequate to keep him upright even in the seated position, and he has to be supported by pillows, leg supports and armrests. He is now prone to sagging to one side of the chair, whereby one of his rigid arms serves as a continuous support, which occasionally leads to nerve damage or fractures. His face also sags to the same side, which can erroneously create the impression that he has suffered a stroke. He is now unable to use his hands and needs to be spoon-fed. He accepts food and drink and opens his mouth automatically. But the actions of chewing, moving the tongue and swallowing are no longer integrated. As a result he keeps the food in his mouth for long periods before he is able to swallow it. Although swallowing is delayed, feeding by mouth remains possible provided the caregiver allows sufficient time, and tries various appetizing nutriments.

It is now very important to prevent and treat complications which can interfere with swallowing, such as thrush, Vincent's angina, or decreased salivation and deglution on account of neuroleptic medication or open mouth breating.

The behavioral disturbances which are prominent and characteristic of the third stage of the illness now mostly subside. The perplexity, the panic, the fear, the agressiveness and the active resistence to the caregiver gradually disappear. The struggle for the preservation of his independence is over. As long as he is still able to walk, he may pace aimlessly up and down for long periods. When he becomes non-ambulatory, he can still pull on his clothes or the bedding, or continuously rub parts of his body. Many expressions of disturbed behavior are now the result of experiences of discomfort. Screaming or lashing out during dressing, bathing or moving the patient are probably caused by pulling on contracted joints, which causes considerable discomfort. Because he cannot move effectively on his own, his rigid limbs may now become molded in the chair, or curl up, reminiscent of the position of a fetus in the womb. Only regular passive stretching of the limbs by the caregiver can prevent total fixation. Abrupt jerking movements of one or more extremities or the entire body may occur, either spontaneously or when he is suddenly taken hold of. Finally, all body movement ceases.

In the scheme of activities of this stage on the following pages, a distinction is sometimes made between phases IVA, IVB, IVC, IVD and IVE, which are indicative of subsequent functional loss. In phase A the patient gradually loses all speech, but can still walk independently. In phase B he can no longer walk, but can still stand (with support) and sit upright. In phase C he cannot sit upright without the support of pillows, but can still move his head. In phase D the latter has also become impossible, but the patient can sometimes still move his arms. In phase E he cannot move his arms any more either. He sometimes opens his eyes, as a reaction to bright light or if he is spoken to in a loud voice. He still reacts to pain, by groans or shrieks. He frequently dozes and yawns when stimulated. Swallowing has become very slow, but the swallowing reflex and the cough reflex often remain intact for a long time, albeit seriously weakened.

What the patient can do himself

as long as he still says a few words spontaneously or walks either independently or with support, he can, provided he does daily active and passive exercises, for about another two and a half years:

√ react to hearing his (given) name called clearly and repeatedly

√ obey extremely simple, very explicit, and often repeated commands, such as: sit down, stand up, walk on, lie down, give, eat, followed by his first name

√ spontaneously use a few standard words to express an emotion

√ repeat an occasional word

√ imitate brief words and sounds

√ turn his head towards someone who stands next to him at eye level and look at him if he is spoken to

√ make laughing sounds if someone standing next to him at eye level laughs

√ get angry if the caregiver gets angry

√ make babbling sounds, such as: ba, ba, ba and repeat this for some time loudly and with increasing rapidity

Intervene observe for, and if necessary prevent

√ almost all awareness of his surroundings and of his own self as an independent person capable of taking action has been lost. Almost the only way in which he can now experience his world at all is in terms of being agreeable or disagreeable

√ he is completely indifferent to objects; he cannot recognize them and they no longer have any significance. He cannot use them in any meaningful way. He now exhibits the primitive behavior of a baby towards objects: grasping, taking hold of and putting them in his mouth

√ repetitive or protracted banging on the armrest of the chair or on the table accompanied by vocal sounds often indicates discomfort (such as with sudden or continuous loud noise, a soiled incontinence system, hunger or thirst, an uncomfortable position, abdominal cramps). Given his condition there exists a multitude of possible causes of discomfort

Partial take-over

√ in order to prevent discomfort for, and agression in the patient, determine beforehand the way in which the patient is to be approached, touched and taken hold of during bathing or dressing. Defensive reactions often occur quickly and can occasionally be violent in character. These reactions are of a primitive defensive nature. They are not intentional, and they protect the patient against anything that may cause potential harm. Everything is potentially dangerous if you are totally helpless

Total take-over

√ remain physically and psychosocially involved with him via auditory and tactile interaction. The patient is now completely oblivious to the fact that he has a body; he has completely lost his body scheme. All the possibilities of making contact with the outside world and with himself have now been lost. Only the caregiver can to some extent still put him in touch with his own body and with the outside world

Attitude

√ discern that the contact of the patient with another person has not been broken, but that it can only be initiated and maintained by that other person, e.g. the caregiver. Up to the end of his life this human being still transmits something to which there can be a meaningful reaction, if the caregiver looks for it, listens, feels and then reflects

√ to give the patient a command should be done in the form of a friendly and persistent request

√ recognize that the urge to move is natural and inherent to every form of life. The urge to move induces the child to walk, but this movement lacks direction. Not until the development of the mental functions does the urge to move come under the control and guidance of the intellect and can it be directed towards an intended goal. In the demented person the natural urge to move emerges again unrestrained on account of the loss of the mental faculties. The caregiver must now guide it, but not impede it

What the   √ give a kiss
patient can   √ imitate some sounds and facial expressions, such as:
do himself   . clack his tongue
                     . loud kissing sound
                     . blow out his cheeks
                     . stick out his tongue
                     . purse his lips
                     . widen his mouth as though tasting something sour
                  √ . shriek, groan, moan or whine

Intervene   √ the patient makes vocal sounds, repeats movements
observe for   over and over again and may experience pleasure from
                      this
                    √ the patient laughs and looks with a certain degree of
                      amazement at the facial mimicry of the caregiver

Total   √ at a short distance from, and on the eye level of
take-over   the patient, evoke and play along with his facial
                      expressions by making sounds and pulling faces which
                      he will mimic

What the patient can do himself

√ move in a slow, hesitant way, without direction, with his head slightly bent, his arms flexed motionless beside or held out in front of his body

√ move from lying down to sitting to standing to remaining standing

√ while standing turn round with small steps in front of a chair, but without managing to sit down

√ walk, when first putting the forefoot and then the heel on the floor

√ get from sitting position to standing in the following way: lean forward, press himself up with both hands on the armrests or seat of the chair and straighten himself to some extent

√ while walking, make grasping movements with his hands

√ on the inclination to fall, grab hold of someone or something in his immediate vicinity

√ sit upright without support

√ spontaneously go from sitting to standing to sitting in a slow and discontinuous motion

√ roll right over from his back to his stomach and vice versa

√ lift up his head from the recumbent position

√ when lying on his stomach, slightly raise his trunk by pressing on his arms

Intervene
observe for,
and if neces-
sary prevent

√ the risk of falling, of contractures of the joints and of
decubitus is now greatly increased

√ the patient can get from lying down to standing, but
not vice versa. This can result in standing for a long
time beside the bed or the chair which may in turn lead
to a fall

√ when trying to roll over from the back to the stomach
in bed, there is the possibility of falling out of bed

√ avoid putting a cervical collar on the patient's neck to
counteract an acquired deformity of his neck. This
usually causes discomfort to the patient. In addition, by
fixing the neck, the muscles of the neck stiffen up,
immobilizing the head

√ there must be no obstacles in his path when he is
walking; in the first instance he tries to
walk round it, but if he is stopped he gets
agitated

√ recognition of the chair as something to sit on is no
longer present. If attempting to sit down, he cannot:
. judge whether he is standing in the right position in
relation to the chair
. place himself in the right position in front of the chair
. judge the distance between his body and the chair

√ as a possible result of the above, when going to sit
down, his bottom may be too far from the seat of the
chair and he lands up on the floor in front of the chair.
He may then break his coccyx or hip, and usually can
no longer sit or lie down without pain

**Partial
take-over**

√ before getting the patient to sit down at the
table, first let him walk a little way

√ when walking is no longer possible, supervise him
when he moves forward or backward in the wheelchair
by pushing his feet, because of the risk of his feet
getting wedged between the footrest and the floor, or
bumping into other people. Give him ample open
space to move about

**Total
take-over**

√ give the patient the necessary freedom of movement and stimulate and facilitate his mobility. This is possible on a platform, on which there is a king size mattress, covered with a ventilated mattress pad. If the patient is no longer able to walk, an air or water mattress, or a vibrating mattress provides an alternative. Such an arrangement has several advantages:
- . more active and passive movement, which helps counteract excessive stiffening of the muscles and joints
- . prevention of decubitus
- . vibration sometimes has a calming effect
- . it is a potential aid in the prevention of immobilizing and painful malformations of the joints (contractures), of pressure neuropathies and of impaired circulation
- . even the severely demented non-ambulant patient often has a life expectation of several more years. He should not be confined to the limits of a bed, which restricts all possible movements which the patient may still have

√ seat the chairbound patient on an anti-decubitus cushion. A seat with soft, nonslip cotton upholstery prevents him from slipping sideways or slumping down and damaging his skin. If the patient sits for long periods on polyvinyl, his skin gets warm and damp and weakens as a result of insufficient ventilation. Evaporation of perspiration and urine in the incontinence system does not occur, which results in skin irritation, particularly in the anal cleft, the groins and the genital area

What the patient can do himself

√ while seated or lying down, make reaching movements with his hands, stimulated by and directed towards visual or tactile impulses

√ stretch out both his arms purposefully towards a person in response to arms stretched out towards him

√ automatically grasp a presented object and hold onto it

√ clasp an offered object in his fist

√ in response to an inviting gesture put an object from his hand into someone else's hand

√ rub and finger an object on all sides with his hand and fingers in an exploring fashion

√ put his hand into a hollow object to grasp an object in the hollow and possibly take it out

√ automatically put something into his mouth which he has in his hand

√ picking, plucking, pulling apart, with both hands

√ move his hand aimlessly through the air, following it with his eyes and reaching out and grasping at real or imaginary objects or persons

grasping is: making hand contact with the outside world and taking hold of that world. Grasping is done with the hand and fingers as a whole. In stage IV it becomes an instinctive behavior, whereby initially visual stimuli still play a part. Still later, grasping only occurs as a reaction to tactile stimulation of the palm of the hand. Grasping involves flexion of the fingers. With strong grasping and pulling, all muscles of the hand and arm become rigid

reaching is: stretching oneself out in space with the intention of making contact with some- thing in the immediate vicinity. It can take place with the whole body, such as for example, with the head and upper part of the body reaching towards food. Reaching requires relaxation of the flexors of the body. When reaching is no longer possible, then there is total stiffening and contractures of the joints quickly occur. By maintaining the reaching action, the total stiffening of the body may be postponed

fingering is: using all fingers together but independently of one another. Fingering requires at least some degree of relaxation of the hand and arm muscles. As long as the patient is able to finger objects, he is able to relax his muscles and overcome the increasing rigidity to some extent

Partial take-over

prevention of dislocation:

√ dislocation of a joint occurs if the maximum load on a joint is seriously exceeded, with the result that the head of the joint is displaced from the socket. The cause may be a fall or a sudden pull on the hand of the patient, such as when the caregiver tries to pull a resisting patient up during the process of moving him from lying down to sitting or from sitting to standing. Dislocation of the shoulder can then occur. Forcing open the mouth of a patient who refuses to open his mouth can result in dislocation of the jaw. In such cases the normal movement capacity and maximal range of motion of a joint is exceeded, causing the head of the joint to be displaced from the socket. Tendons and ligaments are also often torn when a joint is forcefully moved, causing hemorrhage and pain. Dislocation can occur in any joint

Total take-over

√ call in the physician immediately if there are symptoms of a possible dislocation, such as:
. suddenly not being able to move a joint anymore
. groaning or shrieking when the patient is moved and with opening or closing of joints
. local muscle spasm near a joint
. if a joint suddenly exhibits an abnormal form in comparison to the same joint on the other side of the body

What the patient can do himself	√ make searching movements with his hand for an object which has fallen out of his hand and pick it up by chance √ move an object from one hand to the other √ sit opposite the partner and hold an object such as a ball with both hands and join in when the partner moves the object forwards and backwards, up and down or diagonally to the right and left
Intervene observe for, and if necessary prevent	√ if the partner makes abrupt and erratic movements or if there is a difference in tempo between the caregiver and the patient, involuntary muscular tension occurs in the patient, whereby his shoulders, elbows and wrists become temporarily locked. The muscular tension can extend to the rest of the body. As a result he is unable to continue the activity
Partial take-over	√ start the movement of the ball or other object, held by the patient and his partner, slowly and gradually, and let the patient himself from then on determine the rhythm and pace of the to and fro movement as far as possible and adapt to his tempo
Total take-over	√ procure a cloth ball, about 10 inches (25 cm) in diameter, which can be easily grasped and squeezed, with brightly colored figures of about 3 by 1.5 inches (7 by 4 cm) on the surface and with bells on it √ construct objects which rattle when shaken, e.g. a transparent plastic bottle with a well-fitting cap, which the fingers can easily clasp, half full of colored buttons. The rattling sound and the rolling to and fro of the colored contents draws the patient's attention. At the same time, coordinated movements with two hands are stimulated
Attitude	√ realize that recreational activities are now only possible in experiencing pleasure in movement together. The patient is only interested in the object as long as it functions as a means of contact between him and his partner within the game. There is no alternative to human contact with respect to recreational activities in this stage

What the patient can do himself

√ from the supine position hold onto a rope tied in a a fixed loop, and, by means of the partner steering the rope, he can manage to:

. stretch his arms
. move his arms from right to left
. lift his head and trunk
. roll onto the left and right side
. get into the sitting position
. get into the lying down position

Partial take-over

√ with the patient in supine position:

1 let him grasp the loop with both hands and give him the opportunity of getting accustomed to it and fingering it

2 at a distance of 35 inches (80 cm) set a slight movement in motion in the patient by tightening and loosening the rope, until contact and his movements in reaction to the motion of the rope are tangible through the rope

3 walk round the bed with the rope in your hand. By simultaneously tightening or loosening the rope, it is possible to get the patient to perform the movements named above

Total take-over

√ procure about ten feet (four meters) of cotton fiber rope without bulges. Plait the ends together so that the rope forms a non-sliding, fixed loop

√ let the exercises with the rope be accompanied by rhythmic sounds, such as a children's rhyme, humming or music

What the patient can do himself

as long as he can still stand up with support, he can, provided he is stimulated daily:

√ sometimes react with "yes" or "huh" if his given name is clearly and repeatedly called

√ very occasionally still comply with extremely simple, often repeated requests, e.g.: sit, stand, lie down, give, eat

√ produce one or two words spontaneously

√ imitate sounds

√ look at someone who addresses him from close by at eye level

√ grimace and sometimes make laughing sounds when somebody else laughs, who sits close by and at eye level

√ get cross if the caregiver is cross

√ make a repetitive sound reminiscent of babbling, such as: ba, ba, ba for a considerable time

√ give a kiss on an offered mouth or cheek

√ scream in a piercing voice without tonal connection; groan: make a persistent, soft, complaining sound

Intervene observe for, and if necessary prevent

√ protracted and accelerated repetition of parts of words, consisting of a consonant and a vowel, such as "ba, ba, ba", sometimes accompanied by agitated waving movements of the arms and sometimes also of the legs and sometimes with flushing of the face. This behavior often occurs directly after a meal, if he gets emotional and sometimes also when he is addressed. This behavior can be seen as an attempt to talk and a form of making contact

√ protracted soft groans can be a sign of moderate pain or other form of discomfort

√ shrieking piercingly and protractedly is another form of an undifferentiated emotional utterance to attract attention, usually prompted by great distress. Possible causes are: separation, despair, fear, severe pain, anger, discomfort caused by restricted freedom of movement. Thus shrieking calls for immediate attention and search for the possible cause. Protracted shrieking exhausts the patient; once the patient starts, he may not be able to stop because the brain lacks the mechanism to inhibit it

**Total
take-over**

√ create a restful atmosphere with nature sounds
on a disc or tape, such as:
. the surf of the sea
. warbling of birds
. chirruping of crickets
. croaking of frogs
. the wind rustling through the trees
. a running stream
. farm sounds

√ play a disc or tape with classical solo music: flute,
violin, harp

√ try to experiment: individual patients may respond to
different sounds

Attitude

√ shrieking should not be interpreted as intentionally
troublesome behavior which must be 'punished'. The
patient is extremely limited in his possibilities of
expressing and controlling himself. Shrieking calls for a
great deal of energy and if it is carried on for a long
time, it may be caused by a strong, discomfortable
stimulus

What the patient can do himself	√ standing with knees and body bent, when supported by both arms, turn round with small steps
	√ sometimes get from lying down to sitting to standing
	√ in bed, from his own urge to move, get into the sitting posture by pulling himself up by his hands on the safety rail of the bed
	√ get from sitting to standing in a slow and discontinuous movement
	√ sit upright in a (wheel) chair with foot supports, alter his sitting position and pull himself up by his hands if he slips down
	√ roll over from his side to his stomach and sometimes vice versa
	√ in the wheelchair: propel himself forwards or backwards by pushing himself off with his feet
	√ from the recumbent position lift up his head
Intervene observe for, & if necessary prevent	√ patient getting stuck between bed rails and mattress
Partial take-over	√ daily use of massage and exercises, as described in stage IVC
	√ daily provide freedom to, and encourage to move on a king size mattress, as described in stage IVA
Total take-over	√ take him out of doors in his wheelchair and let him touch plants and pets
	√ when taking the wheelchair out of doors, use the safety belt and a calf band to prevent the body tilting forward and the feet from getting wedged

Attitude

√ realize that when the patient on account of the loss of the balance reflexes can no longer sit upright in the chair without being propped up, he may be better off lying on a king size mattress, which is placed on a low platform or on the floor. He then still has some degree of freedom of movement and ample room to move. The mattress can also be put outside in the garden when weather conditions permit. Sitting on a chair is a cultural phenomenon. In many cultures it is perfectly normal to sit or lie on the ground and it is not regarded as inferior or degrading. Being able to move freely on a large comfortable mattress on the floor is preferable to being strapped in a chair

What the patient can do himself

√ when sitting and lying down make reaching and grasping automatic hand movements as a reaction to visual or tactile stimuli from his environment

√ stretch out both his arms to someone as a reaction to arms stretched out to him

√ with stretched arms and unclenched hands make automatic searching movements

√ take hold of an offered object and clasp it in his fist

√ continue to hold an object which fits into his hand for a long time

√ in response to an inviting gesture, put an object from his own hand into someone else's hand

√ pick up and finger an offered object with his hands

√ put his hand in a hollow object such as a box or a jar and grasp and retrieve another object which was put inside

√ move his hand in front of him, following it with his eyes, grasping with his fingers as though to take hold of something

Intervene observe for, and if necessary prevent

√ primitive exploratory behavior in his immediate environment, and self-stimulation are now a last attempt by the patient to get in touch with himself

**Partial
take-over**

√ rope game step by step:

1 induce the grasping action by swinging a rope loop with a diameter of approximately 13 inches (33 cm) loosely to and fro in front of his face, at a distance of 8 inches (21 cm)

2 rub the back of his hand softly, so that the hand opens and subsequently put the rope into it and pull it gently. The grasping reflex is then elicited, which prevents him from letting go of the rope

3 move the rope slowly and gradually and observe the reaction of the patient

4 then move his arm higher, lower and in a circle by means of pulling the rope. Preferably follow the patient's own spontaneous movements

5 in the same way take his other hand and do the exercise with both hands at the same time

6 if the rope is tightly held, stroke the back of his hand from the fingers towards the wrist, so that his hand opens

7 rough movements result in stiffening of the arm, after which it is often impossible to get it moving again. Accompanying the movements by rhythmic singing or music, may enhance the patient's action

**Total
take-over**

√ procure 40 inches (1 meter) of rope (cotton fiber without bulges) and make this into a smooth loop. See stage IVA

√ daily massage and exercises. See for the massage technique IVC, *Purposeful physical contact* 1, 2 and 3

√ when his fingers are not engaged in an activity, put a soft, absorbent, hand-filling object into each of his hands in order to prevent claw-shaped contracture of the fingers

Attitude

√ realize that undifferentiated external stimuli such as light, sound, touching and being touched and internal stimuli, such as pain, can still cause vague general sensations of pleasure or displeasure. These sensations manifest themselves via facial expressions, undifferentiated vocal sounds and rarely by a single word

What the patient can do himself

√ make searching movements with his hand for an object within his visual field

√ move an object from one hand to the other

√ perform a variety of instinctive and reflex self-stimulating movements:

. rub his knees and arms

. scratch his head or other areas

. pluck at something woolly

. suck on a garment or sheet, or on his own fingers

. look intently at and rub the back of his hand

. pull the sleeve of his garment up and down

Intervene observe for, and if neces- sary prevent

√ signs of appreciation during contact with the caregiver

√ he can only distinguish what is close to his eyes, at a distance of approximately one yard (91 cm)

√ he cannot connect the voice of the person speaking to him with that person's face

√ he can still experience tactile stimuli

√ he can sometimes still recognize a familiar voice which he hears every day

Partial take-over

√ with the aid of the requisites listed below (total take-over), the finger movements can be playfully steered by the caregiver

√ a small bucket may lead to grasping and feeling it inside and out

√ a band round the upper arm with bells or figures and objects dangling from a frame lead to grasping, feeling, looking or pulling

√ a glove or cap put on the patient by the caregiver, leads to gripping, stretching, taking off and handling of these objects

√ Velcro figures on a Velcro pad can be pulled off and put back by the patient

**Total
take-over**

√ prevent harmful activities, such as repeated
scratching or abrading, by structurizing the self-
stimulating movements with the aid of the requisites
mentioned below:
- a small plastic bucket with a handle, about 5 inches
  high (13 cm), into which the patient's fist fits easily
- a sweatband, 3 inches wide (8 cm), made of slightly
  elastic material (as used in sport to protect the wrist),
  to which cat's bells have been attached
- a similar armband with colorful fabric or plastic
  figures tacked onto it
- a righthand and a lefthand cotton glove, with for
  example a clown's face
- a jockey cap
- a Velcro pad with matching colorful Velcro figures
- a frame with square corners, to be attached to chair
  or bed, with objects fastened to it by a string so that
  they dangle

√ look for possible irritating skin conditions as a cause of
scratching

√ avoid restraining his hand whenever possible

√ prevent the patient from putting objects into his mouth

What the patient can do himself

as long as he can actively keep his head and trunk upright after being sat up in the chair, he can – provided he is activated and passively exercised daily:

√ react with a grunt or sometimes with "yes" if his given name is clearly and repeatedly called out

√ look at someone if he is spoken to from close by

√ smile at the caregiver, if the latter smiles

√ get angry and resistant when the caregiver acts irritated

√ imitate simple vocal sounds

√ make a repetitive babbling sound in an attempt to talk

√ kiss an offered mouth or cheek

√ scream and shriek penetratingly and with persistence

√ groan and moan with persistence

√ when kept standing upright, by supporting him under both his arms, he can bear the weight of his own body for a short time

√ before moving stretch out his arms

√ hold onto the caregiver firmly with both hands

√ in a wheelchair with foot supports sit upright and move the chair forwards and backwards via pushing or pulling movements with his feet

√ roll over from his side to his back or his stomach

√ lift up his head from the recumbent position

√ sitting and lying down make automatic reaching and grasping movements with his hands in response to visual or tactile stimuli

√ stretch out one or both arms in someone's direction

√ reach out with his hand(s) for an offered object

√ grasp an object which fits into his hand and keep it in his fist for some time

√ make searching movements with his hand for a visible object which has fallen out of his hand

√ move an object from one hand into the other

√ finger an object held in his hand

√ in response to an inviting gesture put something out of his hand into someone else's hand

√ put his hand into a hollow object, reach for another object that is inside, and take it out

Intervene
observe for,
and if neces-
sary prevent

√ sudden buckling of the knees while standing
   unsupported, leading to a fall
√ slumping down or sliding down when changing his
   sitting position
√ continual inefficient shifting of position in the chair, as
   a result of which decubitus can occur on his seat and
   elbows; falls, decubitus and sliding down in his chair
   can be prevented by putting him in a reclining chair
   with his legs supported in the horizontal position.
   Restraining the patient can thus be avoided

**Total
take-over**

√ *General instructions for massage*
- for the hand massage, the patient sits upright, with his
  head supported and with his knees bent at an angle of
  45 degrees. The caregiver-massager sits opposite the
  patient
- apply a moisturizing and lubricating cream or lotion at
  room temperature while massaging; the hands glide
  over the skin more easily and the condition of the skin
  is improved
- for the foot massage (see Ch. IV, stage IIIB, Foot Care)
  the patient leans backwards, in a half-sitting position
  with his legs supported in the horizontal position and
  his feet projecting slightly over the edge
- see that the nails of the massaging fingers do not press
  into the patient's skin
- massage by slowly pressing, rubbing, stroking and
  turning the patient's fingers
- observe the patient's face for expressions of pleasure or
  displeasure
√ *Handmassage*
- take the patient's hand, with the back of the hand
  uppermost, in the palm of your own hand
- place the fingers of your own hands under the fingers
  of the patient's hand and your thumbs on top of the
  patient's fingers
- using your two thumbs, softly knead the fingers and
  thumb of the patient, working from the fingertips to
  the base of the fingers and between the fingers

√ *Massage of the back of the hand*
- place the palm of the patient's hand on his knee or on your own knee
- put the palm of your hand on the back of the patient's hand
- now make slowly rotating, lightly pressing movements

√ *Wrist and arm massage*
- enclose the patient's wrist with your fingers and thumbs
- make kneading and rotating movements over the wrists, upper and under arm with both hands in opposite directions

√ *Hand-wrist exercise*
- support the patient's elbow with one hand
- with the other hand grasp the patient's fingers
- bend the hand gently and gradually downwards at the wrist
- hold the patient's wrist in one hand
- put your own hand and fingers against those of the patient
- press the hand gently and slowly upwards

√ *Finger exercise*
- press softly on the phalanxes
- gently stretch finger for finger and massage at the same time

√ *Wrist-elbow exercise*
- take hold of his hand at the sides with your two hands
- gradually stretch the patient's arm
- make slow rotating movements to the left and to the right with his hand

√ *Wrist-finger exercise*
- put the palm of your own hand against the palm of the patient's hand
- put your fingers between the patient's fingers
- subsequently make slow, repeated bending and stretching movements with your own fingers

√ *Arm massage*
- take hold of his upper arm between your two hands
- pull your hands very slowly along his arm right to the fingertips and hold them for a short time

- this massage and the exercises can also be applied to the feet and legs

Attitude

√ realize that the contact sensation is the most elementary of the senses, the first to be present to the new born and the last to disappear in the demented person. It is the only means that the patient still has at his disposal, to communicate with the world. Through the sensation of contact he can experience the world mainly as pleasurable or as disagreeable. His skin is now virtually the only sense organ left to him. Without being touched by another person, the patient is now completely isolated. It is only by means of another person's hands that this isolation can be temporarily penetrated

√ much can still be achieved by purposeful touching, such as in massage: rest and relaxation of a continuously screaming patient are often achieved by it

What the patient can do himself

√ make self-stimulating movements with his fingers:
  . rub his knees and arms
  . rub or scratch his head or other parts of his body
  . pull fluff off wooly fabric
  . suck on a garment or bedsheet

√ move his hand in front of him following it with his eyes. He is unable to recognize his hand as his own

√ with his hand or fist bang on the table board or the armrest of the chair; often for long periods and accompanied by vocal sounds

Total take-over

√ perform the various activities described in stage IV together with the patient:
- stimulate his emotions by means of making sounds with your mouth and facial expressions
- give him freedom of movement by laying him on a king size mattres, and stimulate him to move or move him passively
- stimulate him to make hand/arm movements by means of a rope, ball or other object which is held by both patient and caregiver
- create a calming environment by playing tapes with soft music or sounds of nature
- structurize the existing self-stimulating finger movements by means of requisites as discussed in this chapter
- take him out of doors in the wheelchair

What the patient can do himself

as long as the patient, sitting with support for his trunk and his back, and his arms supported by armrests, is able to actively move his head, he can, on condition that he is daily activated and passively exercised, spontaneously but not on command:

√ sometimes react when his given name is clearly called out by looking at his partner

√ look at someone who speaks to him from close by

√ smile at the caregiver, if the latter begins to laugh or speaks to him affectionately

√ make a repetitive babbling sound

√ sometimes give a kiss on an offered mouth or cheek

√ scream for long periods of time; groan and make protracted soft moaning sounds during each exhalation

√ slightly turn, stretch and bend his head

√ move his head-trunk as an entity, rocking forward and back to the back of the chair by shifting the center of gravity of the body

√ when being moved, keep his head in one line with his body

√ roll over from his side to about halfway onto his back (but not in reverse)

Intervene observe for, and if necessary prevent

√ vague, non-discriminative sensations brought about by various stimuli from the outside world, such as movement, light and sound, gradually lose their significance for the patient. But sensations of cold, heat, painful pressure or gentle stroking and warmth continue to exist for a long time. The patient experiences them mainly as pleasurable or diagreeable. He reacts to pleasurable sensations with a smile, an expression of content, by stretching his arms or opening his hands. He reacts to disagreeable sensations by withdrawing his arms or legs, groaning or shrieking. When he experiences something as being pleasant, then he is calm and has a relaxed and peaceful expression on his face, which comes about for instance if he is touched caressingly

√ when he is sitting down, the hollow of his back together with the neighbouring parts of the right and left trunk, must be firmly supported

√ lengthy periods of passively sitting with his
knees bent cause slipping down in the (rocking) chair
and the increased pressure from shifting position causes
decubitus on his seat and impairs circulation in the legs

√ never impede the seated rocking motion by
immobilizing the patient by means of a restraint band
or in other ways

**Total
take-over**

√ transmit feelings of affection by talking to him
in a friendly way and by stroking:
- putting out a hand to him and rubbing the back of his
hand
- lightly squeezing his upper and lower arm
- rubbing his back and shoulders
- putting your fingers caressingly through his hair like a
comb, thereby softly massaging the scalp
- taking his head in one or both of your hands, pressing
it against you, putting the flat of your hand on his head
and making softly pressing, rotating movements

√ *skin massage*
- after bathing rub a skin-protecting cream or lotion into
the body and gently scratch and tap with your fingertips

√ *scalp massage*
- stand behind the patient, let one hand rest loosely on
his forehead to support his head and to prevent the
neck muscles from becoming tensed
- use the index, middle and ring fingers for the massage
- massage by means of lightly touching, with short up
and down movements; from the crown, over the
middle, to the occipital area. Then along the base of
the skull to above the ears. Avoid pulling his hair
during the massage by lifting your fingers when moving
from one massage point to another

√ *neck and back massage*
- stand behind the sitting patient and slowly massage his
neck, shoulders and back with rotating movements of
the hands. This massage, when regularly applied, may
to some extent alleviate the rigidity of the neck and
back muscles which causes the body to curve

**What the
patient can
do himself**

*sitting with his head and back supported, make automatic
movements as a reaction to certain visual or tactile
stimuli from his immediate surroundings:*
√ clasp an object in his fist and hold it for a short time
√ put an object from his hand into his mouth
√ make self-stimulating movements with his fingers: rub
his arms; scratch his head; suck a garment or bedsheet;
look at and rub one finger over one particular spot on
the back of his hand
√ move his hand in front of him, following it with his
eyes (he does not recognize his hand as his own any
more and may try to grasp it with his other hand)

Intervene
observe for,
and if neces-
sary prevent

√ when he can no longer remain seated upright on his
own, (i.e. without supports), and his trunk tilts
forwards, backwards or sideways, he can also no longer
change his sitting position or pull himself up if he slips
down. The result of this uncontrollable sitting posture
is often a rocking movement, forwards and backwards
with his head-trunk as an entity. He is unable to move
his limbs independently to shift his position

**Partial
take-over**

√ seat the patient during the day in a reclining
chair on wheels, and with adjustable support for his
legs and from the legs up to his head. In this type of
chair the patient can both sit (with bent knees) and lie
(with his legs stretched). His position can then
regularly be changed, which prevents him from
becoming fixed in the 'sitting on a chair' posture

**Total
take-over**

√ perform the various activities on the patient,
as mentioned in stage IV:
- massage/exercises of his body, head, hands, feet
- stimulation of his facial expressions by making noises
with your mouth and pulling faces
- provide freedom of movement and encouragement to
move (or move him passively) on the king size mattress
- let him move his hands and arms via a rope loop or
hoop

- provide a restful environment with calming sounds
- stimulate his remaining visual abilities by hanging a bright object, which moves with the air current, on a frame attached to the chair or bed
- provide a pacifier on a ring on which the patient can suck or put a clean moist washcloth in his hand for the same purpose
- take him out of doors in the wheelchair

What the patient can do himself

when, supported in the sitting or lying position, he can no longer hold up or lift up his head on his own, he can, provided he is daily stimulated and passively exercised:

√ perceive bright light and loud sound as pleasant or unpleasant

√ sigh deeply and sometimes catch his breath, yawn

√ if caressed on his cheek, direct his head to the side of the caressed cheek

√ scream and shriek, groan, make protracted soft moaning sounds

√ clasp an object in his hand if it comes in contact with the palm of his hand

√ move his mouth towards an object which touches his lips and grip it with his lips

√ sometimes move his hands in the direction of his mouth or his pubic area

√ if the corner of his mouth or the skin round his mouth are touched, make searching and sucking movements in the direction of the object in contact

√ suck an object the caregiver puts in his mouth

observe for, and if necessary prevent

√ when he can no longer hold his head up on his own, he can be placed in a reclining chair as described in stage IVD with the back tilted backwards at an angle of 45 degrees, with his legs in the horizontal position and the hollow of his back and adjacent parts of his left and right side supported. It is to be observed that:

- the head, neck and trunk are now totally passive

- the arms are not stretched any more

- his fingers still sometimes grasp an object and put it in the mouth

- the legs and feet become involuntarily crossed over one another, or

- the knees are usually pressed against one another

√ most motion now gradually ceases. Sudden, brief, vapid jerking movements of one or more extremities or of the entire body may occur, either spontaneously or provoked by stimuli from the environment, such as loud sounds or a sudden touch

Total
take-over

√ always support the head and trunk as one entity while moving the patient from the sitting position to lying down and vice versa. His neck is often immovable on account of the continuously tensed neck muscles

√ when the patient is in the sitting position, his head, trunk and legs must be supported, since otherwise his head/trunk will tilt to one side, mostly the same side. Not infrequently a contracture of the head occurs in one direction

√ frequently change his position. Lying for any length of time on the same side or on his back is painful and causes successively irritation of the skin, blisters, a sore and ultimately necrosis (decubitus) on the parts of the body most exposed to pressure: back of the head, ears, shoulders, hips, bottom, inside and outside of the knees and ankles

What the patient can do himself

√ as long as he can still walk, step under the shower head in a shower cabin without a bath tub or a high threshold. He can no longer step into the bath tub

√ express feelings of discomfort by:
. shrieking
. groaning
. clutching someone else, the chair or his bed
. cover a part of his body with his hand in a gesture of modesty
. withdraw an arm or leg
. assume a huddled up posture

Encourage

√ as long as he can still walk: guide him to the bathroom and the shower or give the encouragement by means of inviting gestures

Intervene observe for, and if necessary prevent

√ having to be washed all over is confusing and can be frightening, because the patient:
- does not understand the reason for the caretaker's presence nor his objective
- cannot orientate himself to his own body any more during the washing activities (or any other activities)
- can no longer adapt his body to the space surrounding him, i.e., the shower, bath or bed
- does not understand why the caregiver constantly moves his body into various positions, such as holding up, bending and stretching his arms and legs, putting his legs apart and touching the pubic area

√ loss of balance and falling. Although the patient initially is able to stand and sit with support:
- his body does not remain in balance for longer periods of time
- his arms are usually stretched out and his hands make grasping movements
- he is unable to recognize a potential source of support when he threatens to lose his balance
- the patient becomes restless on account of the uncomfortable position, gets irritated and is prone to fall

√ restlessness and resistance to washing can cause a fall
√ an increasingly rigid posture is to be seen, whereby through relative immobility the joints are easily prone to contractures. When a joint becomes permanently fixed, with either complete or partial loss of the passive range of motion, a contracture exists. This is usually brought about by an abnormal tone in the muscles which move the joint, in combination with inactivity of the joint. Once a contracture is permanent, there is always deformity of the joint. Contractures greatly impair the quality of life of the patient and must be prevented at all costs. The body can then no longer be brought into the normal sitting and lying position. Malformations of the joints occur, such as:

- a permanently fixed position of the head, caused by protracted leaning over to one side
- the arms being permanently flexed in the elbows and turned inwards, pressed against the body or held away from it
- the wrists being permanently flexed and turned in the direction of the permanently flexed thumbs, with the fingertips pressed into the palm of the hands
- the vertebral column being permanently curved sideways in an arch, causing the lowest rib and the top of the pelvis to touch one another
- the trunk being permanently bent forward and the head in an abnormal position
- the hips and knees being permanently flexed and the legs crossed, whereby they can no longer be moved apart
- the ankles being permanently fixed at an angle of 90°, or turned in the direction of the big toe with the forefeet stretched downwards
- a permanent fixation of the body in the 'sitting on the chair position', or involuted, and resembling the fetus posture, as a result of which it is impossible for the patient to lie stretched out on his back. The knees and ankles are often painfully pressed against each other in this position

**Total
take-over**

√ investigate which (component) actions and which movements give rise to expressions of pain or anxiety, e.g.:
- when being moved; by pulling on the joints, for
  example the shoulders.
- by shearing force on the skin
- by spreading the legs or stretching and bending the
  extremities
- by turning and bending his head

√ every day *before* washing the patient, judge his mood
and mobility and identify possible complicating
circumstances. Take action accordingly:
- determine the place for the washing activity: shower,
  bath or bed
- put the requisites out ready and regulate the room
  temperature, which should be 78° F (25° Centigrade)
- take safety measures (e.g., chair, nonslip mat in shower)
- if necessary, call in the help of a second aide
- estimate the duration of the total activity and take
  measures accordingly to ensure that you can perform
  the activity without being disturbed
- approach, accompany and move the patient in a quiet
  and secure atmosphere

√ *during* the specifically oriented activity:
- use a hand shower instead of the overhead shower
- adapt the washing actions to the body postures and
  movements of the patient
- regularly inspect the patient's body for abnormalities
  of the skin and joints
- adjust the pace of all necessary actions to the mood
  and tempo of the patient

√ when the patient can no longer walk on his own,
use is made of a patient's lift to transfer him from the
bed into the bathtub or into the stool and vice versa.
Some points to be noted in the use of such a lift are:
- the lift is often frightening for the patient, who is
  unable to understand that this appliance has been
  chosen on account of efficiency and sparing pain
- use two people to fix the hammock and operate the
  lift

- before beginning to move him, first raise him slightly above the mattress and check whether his back, legs, arms and head are well supported
- raise, move and lower the patient slowly, so that he does not swing to and fro, and remain visible to him and talk to him

√ *after* the washing activity: assess the physical and psychological situation and adjust the next activity, dressing, accordingly

√ when attempting to reposition the patient, lift him instead of shoving him

√ during his caring activities the caregiver must avoid wearing jewellery, such as rings which can damage the skin, and earrings or chains which the patient can clutch. Long nails are unpractical

points for particular attention in caring for a patient with contractures of the joints:

√ as a result of the contractures he is totally invalid, unable to move at all and dependent on the caregiver for even the slightest change in position

√ fear and pain aggravate the formation of contractures

√ corrective treatment is no longer feasable, because the patient does not understand the purpose and is unable to cooperate with the therapist. The sometimes accompanying pain of the therapy is also counterproductive

√ an abnormal fixed position of the head impedes it being lifted up, laid down, turned and moved up and down and to and fro and causes premature loss of functioning

√ a permanently extended, flexed or rotated neck may contribute to stenosis of the cervical canal, with compression of the spinal cord, and result in premature loss of ambulation

√ an abnormally fixed position of the head can seriously impede swallowing

Take care:
- carefully observe the patient's facial and vocal expressions; they are the only indicators of physical distress or comfort

- when moving the head/neck/trunk as one entity, support the head. Do not attempt to turn the head separately
- support the head with pillows in such a way that it is comfortably resting. This is particularly important if the neck is permanently bent through increased muscular tension

√ a fixed posture of the arms impedes the mobility of the shoulder and elbow joints

Take care:
- do not try to forcibly stretch the joints of the shoulder and elbow during the care actions. Instead, slowly and gradually try to stretch them, at the same time massaging the extensor muscles of the upper arm
- when the patient is in the sitting position, support the armpits and forearms with pillows

√ with a permanently flexed position of the wrist and the fingers, the fingertips continuously press into the palm of the hand

Take care: good hand hygiene is essential:
- keep the palm of the hand dry after cleaning it
- cut the nails short and keep them clean
- check on pressure sores on the palm of the hand and between the fingers
- put a roll of soft, absorbent material, for example a washcloth, into the patient's hands, and pads of similar material in between the fingers

√ with the vertebral column permanently bent sideways (scoliosis), skin irritation and local pain can occur on account of pressure and chafing of the lowest rib against the rim of the pelvis

Take care: put a piece of flannel or lint between the rib and the rim of the pelvis

√ when the hips are permanently turned inwards, the legs are permanently crossed

Take care:
- prevent decubitus on the inside of the knees and the outside of the ankles by placing a cushion pad between them and wrapping the ankles in protective material
- prevent skin irritation and eczema in the groins and the genital area, resulting from permanent hyperflexion

of the hips, by blow-drying the skin after drying it with a towel. Spread and stretch the legs a little, carefully and gradually

√ with a vertebral column which is bent forward in the pelvic area, skin irritation can occur in the stomach crease and the groins

√ with a forefoot which is stretched downwards there is very little space between the toes

Take care:
- prevent the occurrence of skin irritation by gentle cleansing and blow-drying of the skin. Thereafter apply a lubricating skin lotion
- use heel protectors to prevent decubitus

√ with deformity and fixation of the body, the skin becomes still more atrophic on account of the diminished skin circulation and compression neuropathy. Every place on the skin is then vulnerable if it is subjected to pressure

Take care:
- frequently turn the patient over onto his other side
- put cushion pads between the leg and knees
- apply a lubricating skin lotion after washing the patient and in the evening

Attitude
√ all motions are now undifferentiated, are no longer intentional, and are often elicited by the actions of another person. Most movements are now basic motions: either grasping movements or defensive movements, pulling something towards him or pushing it away. He can no longer put his body into operation, and consequently the patient is no longer capable of cooperating either actively or passively with the caregiver

What the patient can do himself

√ spontaneously, but not on command, spit out something unpleasant in the mouth

√ slowly drink and swallow

Intervene observe for, and if necessary prevent

√ inflammation of the mucous membrane of the mouth (stomatitis) or tongue (glossitis) or gums (gingivitis). Some possible causes:

- diminished resistance because of malnutrition
- fluid depletion as a result of an infectious illness (such as influenza)
- dehydration of the oral cavity on account of too little intake of fluid, or too dry air and a constantly open mouth
- decrease in production of saliva, also as a side effect of medication
- badly fitting or damaged dentures
- inadequate oral hygiene
- constant breathing through the mouth on account of nasal congestion or weakness of the facial muscles

**Total
take-over**

√ regular inspection of the oral cavity. The consequences of poor oral hygiene can be recognized by:
- persisting bad breath
- red, swollen and easily bleeding gums which are sensitive to pressure
- dirty yellow gray spots on the mucous membrane, the tonsils, the tongue, the palate and inner side of the lips. All these signs are indicative of Vincent's angina. They result in difficulty with swallowing
- blisters on the edge of the lips and on the mucous membrane, which change into painful ulcers, are indicative of herpes
- white patches on a reddish inflamed mucous membrane of the oral cavity, tonsils and gingiva, accompanied by difficulty and pain in swallowing are indicative of thrush (candidiasis).

√ consult the physician or dentist with the symptoms mentioned above. Dental treatment is very difficult in stage IV unless given under general anesthesia

√ people with colds or infections should be kept away from the patient. When the caregiver has a cold, he must see to it that he washes his hands frequently when caring for the patient and avoid blowing his nose or sneezing or coughing in the patient's vicinity

√ the caregiver should always wash his own hands before and after cleaning the patient's mouth, and use disposable material

√ let the patient drink three pints of fluid per 24 hours and give mint tea for fresh breath

√ clean the patient's mouth twice a day, for instance with a lemon flavored glycerine swab. Do not use a disinfectant mouthwash, because the patient can no longer spit it out

√ keep the patient's lips lubricated day and night

√ to have the patient open his mouth, approach it with the swab, or gently stroke the lips. The mouth can be briefly kept open by inserting a soft object such as a rolled up moist washcloth between his teeth and holding it by the end with one hand

What the patient can do himself

√ the patient can no longer purposefully or even passively join in the actions of the caregiver during the process of being dressed. He can express and react to discomfort by:
. groaning
. shrieking
. clasping the other person, the chair or the bed
. grasping for and holding onto a garment
. withdraw an arm or leg
. assume a huddled up posture
. lash out at the caregiver
. if the palm of his hand is touched, close his hand and draw his arm towards him in a reflex action

Intervene observe for, and if necessary prevent

√ discomfort in the patient while he is being dressed: the process of being dressed can be uncomfortable and frightening, because the patient is at the mercy of the caregiver during an activity which is totally incomprehensible to him, and also because the garments are continually changing their form. He is not able to:
- adjust to the tempo of the caregiver
- assume the required changes of position of his limbs, such as: bending, stretching and turning
- follow the proceeding of the movements of the caregiver and adjust his posture and motions accordingly
- follow the progress of the dressing activity

√ the caregiver can facilitate dressing the patient by sitting opposite him at the patient's eye level during the procedure, because:
- it promotes contact
- the limbs do not have to be raised or pulled unnecessarily, which means less risk of pain and anxiety
- it encourages spontaneous movement which can be made use of to facilitate dressing

√ the regulation of the patient's temperature is often disturbed on account of the abnormal functioning of the temperature regulation center in the brain (in the hypothalamus). Hyperthermia is an abnormally high body temperature, i.e., 106° F (41° C), usually as a result of hot weather, in combination with insufficient fluid intake. Dehydration (see also Chapter IV page 190) is commonly present with hypernatremia (increased sodium concentration of the blood). Initially the patient may exhibit increased confusion with hallucinations, rapidly followed by unconsciousness and seizures. The skin is hot and dry, the pulse is rapid and the blood pressure is low. Immediate treatment is required. When the patient survives, paralysis of all extremities may result. .

√ if a quilt is used instead of blankets in a damp, warm environment the body heat accumulates under the quilt. Through a decrease in the heat emission of the body, as happens in the absence of transpiration, heat congestion and restlessness occur because the patient is unable to remove the quilt

√ hypothermia: undercooling of the body with a body temperature below 95° F (35° C) through too low temperature of the environment easily occurs on account of the disturbed function of the temperature regulation center in the brain; the reduction of the protective subcutaneous layer of fat (malnourishment); reduced physical activity, especially in the case of restraint for longer periods; diminished shivering and certain medications, in particular neuroleptics, which affect the temperature regulation center in the brain and which may cause increased rigidity and hypokinesia (abnormally diminished muscular activity). Hypothermia in these patients may already occur with a temperature of 60° F. Signs and complications of hypothermia are: decreased activity, drowsiness, stupor, increased muscular rigidity, slow pulse, skin cold to touch (also the trunk), dehydration, seizures, pneumonia and cardiac arrest. Hypothermia is a medical emergency

√ with rapid cooling off the patient feels uncomfortable, muscular rigidity occurs which makes it more difficult to bathe and dress him

**Total
take-over**

√ slowly and gradually move the patient's arms and
legs into the desired position. If the caretaker passively
moves the patient's limbs erratically, such as putting the
patient's hand into the armhole with a rapid movement
and pulling the garment on further in fairly high
tempo, the patient becomes rigid and agitated. Even
though the patient does try to follow the dressing
movements and join in through the movements of the
caregiver, the difference in direction and speed of
motion between the caregiver and the patient prevents
this and evokes involuntary muscular tension in the
patient. His shoulder, elbow and wrist become
temporarily locked. Not infrequently the provoked
muscular tension spreads to the rest of the body

√ putting on a sweater, shirt or dress:
- first put the garment over the patient's head
- subsequently put your own hand into one of the
  sleeves via the collar
- push your hand through to the lower edge of the
  sweater, so that it becomes visible (in doing this the
  sleeve rolls up over the caregiver's arm)
- now take the patient's hand in your own hand,
  meanwhile softly massaging the palm of his hand,
  which leads to the occurrence of the grasping reflex
  and the patient keeps hold of the care- giver's hand
- now pull the patient's hand, guided by your own
  hand, through the sleeve
- in order to break loose from a strong grasping reflex,
  massage the back of the hand
- repeat the same actions with the other sleeve

√ the same technique can be used in putting on trousers

√ prevent excessive cooling off during washing or
dressing by:
- putting all requisites for changing and washing ready
  within reach
- briefly preheat the incontinence system (i.e., the
  disposable adult briefs)
- always wash the patient with warm water
- see that cotton, linen or woolen clothes are worn,

which provide good insulation, while allowing better skin ventilation

- see that long trousers or panty hose are worn. because there is almost always a draught at floor level
- see that long underwear is worn so that there is no uncovered area between trousers/skirt and blouse/sweater. It is important to keep the lower part of the body covered because the stomach area is the warmest place in the body
- adjust clothing to the ambient temperature and cover both his legs and his head when going outside. Protect him from wind and sun
- immediately change the wet disposable briefs

Attitude   √ see that the patient does indeed wear the clothes he has brought with him and which are intended for him

√ realize that a neglected outward appearance often leads to the patient being less respectfully treated by his environment

√ realize that regular variation in his clothes, matching outfits and well-cared for, clean, well-fitting clothing is an expression of a respectful and caring attitude towards the patient

What the patient can do himself

√ *as long as he is still able to say about half a dozen different intelligible words in the course of an average day, either spontaneously or when being spoken to, and walks independently, he can, on condition that he has daily activities and passive exercises, spontaneously but not on command:*
  . sit upright and to some extent change his
  . position in the chair while eating
  . use both arms and hands sitting at the table
  . reach for an object at arm's length, search with his hand for the exact position of the object, grasp it, pick it up, hold it and bring it to his mouth
  . leave his plate on the table while eating
  . scoop up solids or semi-solids with a spoon
  . slowly put a spoon with thick soup or solid food into his mouth with occasional spilling
  . eat from the plate with the spoon
  . put food in his mouth with his fingers
  . empty his plate with his hands and tongue
  . drink from a glass or mug which he holds with both hands
  . drink through a straw
√ slowly chew and swallow puréed and minced food, swallow liquids
√ spontaneously, but not on command, spit out food
√ automatically open his mouth on seeing a spoon or mug approaching his mouth
√ sometimes say 'thank you' at the appropriate moment
√ sometimes excuse himself with a word or gesture for audibly burping

Intervene

√ finding the food on his plate may become more difficult because of impaired depth vision and convergence
√ chewing and swallowing of food goes very slowly and it is difficult for him to remove hard pieces of food with his tongue because:
  - the complex mechanism of chewing, tongue and swallowing motions is now less coordinated and each of these separate motions now has its own tempo

- the motions of the tongue are no longer purposefully steered and have slowed down
- the patient cannot determine the location of the food in his mouth, so that he is unable to remove it with his tongue (such as food stuck to the palate)

√ the ability to chew remains intact, albeit it with less efficiency, until he is no longer able to hold his head upright

√ aspiration of food: the patient is unable to actively expel food which has got into the windpipe. Nor does he understand the encouragement to cough and breathe deeply afterwards, which is needed to remove the food that is lodged in the windpipe, and completely depends on the efficiency of his cough reflex. Aspirated food and liquids may find their way into the lungs. Recurrent aspiration can result in a very persistent inflammation of the pulmonary tissue; this 'aspiration or chemical pneumonitis' is often difficult to treat, and can form a serious threat to the patient's life. Difficulty with breathing occurs within a few hours, but fever often does not occur until several days after the aspiration, when a bacterial infection is superimposed

observe for, and if necessary prevent

Partial take-over

√ allow him ample time to eat

√ let the patient eat at his own tempo, however slow it may be

√ if necessary steer his hand with the fork or spoon in the scooping position to the food on the plate. Let him put the fork or spoon into his mouth himself and return it to the plate

√ if necessary guide his hand to the drinking glass or mug on the table or guide his hand with the mug to his mouth

Total take-over

√ see that there is a restful atmosphere during the meal without any distraction

√ sit down when helping the patient with eating and drinking for the following reasons:
- to be able to see each other's facial expressions; this promotes contact and bears witness to interest in the patient
- the patient need not turn or bend his head back with every bite. Older people often have arthrosis of the cervical vertebra and partial blockage of the carotid arteries; pain, giddiness and nausea can occur when the head is bent back
- the caregiver is better able to steer his own hand movements
- the caregiver is able to observe the patient's mouth and determine whether it is empty before he takes the next mouthful - this diminishes the chances of choking

√ provide properly prepared aliments to prevent aspiration of liquids and food. The aliments must:
- be free of coarse grains, threads, skin, peel, hard pieces and not have a crumbly structure
- be free of substances which excessively stimulate the mucous membrane of the mouth such as: carbonated drinks; too much salt; too sour, sweet, bitter or too spicey food
- even consistency: contain sufficient fluid, be smooth, fine, puréed; smooth cream soup; slightly creamy drinks etc.
- avoid food and drinks which the patient shows an aversion to, so as to avoid retching
- if excessive production of mucus occurs, replace milk or milk dishes by expectorants, such as unsweetened fruit juice
- the temperature of food and drink influences the appetite. Spitting out, coughing, panting and unexpected movements caused by too hot food can lead to aspiration

√ when helping the patient to eat:
- put small quantities on the spoon

- wait until the patient has emptied his mouth before spooning up the next mouthful
- wait until the patient's mouth is oriented to the spoon, his attention has been drawn to it and he opens his mouth of his own accord before putting the spoon into his mouth
- do not force him to open his mouth. By caressing or lightly tapping his cheek, the corner of his mouth or his upper lip his mouth usually opens of its own accord
- put solid food into his mouth in such a way that it does not stick to his palate. He is unable to remove it with his tongue, and retching occurs
- never force food on the patient

What the patient can do himself

as long as he can still stand when supported, he can, on condition he is daily activated and passively exercised, spontaneously but not on command:

√ during the meal remain sitting upright and change position in his chair

√ using his fingers take food from his plate and put it in his mouth

√ sometimes hold the drinking cup with both hands while drinking

√ sitting at the table search for an object with his hands, grasp it, pick it up, hold it, pull it towards him and let it go again after an indefinite period

√ slowly chew and swallow puréed food

√ reject food by spitting it out

√ lick; suck

√ sip liquids through a straw

√ open his mouth automatically when being spoon fed

√ cough when aspirating food or liquids

Intervene observe for, and if necessary prevent

√ in the event of aspiration of food , it can happen that after the coughing ceases, food or liquids have gone down into the windpipe and the lungs, with the result that a branch of the windpipe becomes blocked, part of the lung collapses and inflammation may develop (aspiration pneumonia). After a case of aspiration, continue to observe the patient for several days and report any symptoms which may occur, such as cough, fever, tightness of the chest, rapid, shallow and difficult respiration, refusing food or rapid pulse

**Partial
take-over**

prevention of aspiration

√ correct posture for eating:
  . sitting upright against the back of the chair and with
    support for the feet (see also stage III)
  . bedridden patients: sitting upright, head, back and
    arms supported
    support the sitting patient in such a way that he is
    prevented from slipping down or tilting his trunk to
    one side
  . elevate the head of the bed about 8 inches (20 cm)
    above the feet, when the patient is predisposed to
    aspiration

√ Use of medication:
  . certain medications, such as sedatives or neuroleptics
    can partly be the cause of difficulties with chewing,
    swallowing, a dry mouth and drowsiness, resulting in
    an increased predisposition to aspiration
  . mixing medicine through a whole portion of food or
    drink can lead to retching, spitting out or vomiting
    and inefficient absorption of the medication

**Total
take-over**

√ assistence with eating:
  . put a plate with small ready-to-eat morsels, small
    portions at a time, in front of him and let him eat on
    his own as much as possible
  . avoid giving fluids when the head is bent backwards or
    forwards
  . give small amounts of fluid which can be swallowed in
    one gulp

What the patient can do himself

as long as he can actively keep his head and trunk upright after being put into the sitting position in his chair, and on condition that he is engaged in the activity and passively exercised daily, he can:

√ sometimes take hold of a mug by one or both handles, pick it up when it is handed to him and drink from the lip

√ occasionally eat food with his hands

√ eat from the spoon which the caregiver brings to his mouth

√ react to the movement of the spoon towards his mouth by opening his mouth

√ chew and swallow slowly

√ push food out of his mouth with his tongue

√ cough when aspirating food or liquids

Intervene observe for, and if necessary prevent

√ aspiration of food, whereby food or liquids get into the larynx or windpipe and are not coughed up, with the result that the windpipe is partially or sometimes totally blocked. Labored wheezy inhalation occurs with contraction of the muscles above the collarbone. In the case of total blockage, the face becomes successively red, pale and blue. Immediate application of the Heimlich maneuver (see section *total take-over*) can save his life. At the first signs of choking immediately call in help and begin with the Heimlich maneuver without delay

Partial take-over

√ ways to prevent aspiration of food are:

. never force the patient to eat or drink. He is unable to swallow or empty his mouth on command

. do not let him drink through a straw

. do not give him candy or chewing gum: he can no longer suck it, bite through it or spit it out

. do not give him toast or cookies; crumbs irritate the throat and can expand in the fluid of the windpipe

. check the condition of his mouth daily; look out for loose or missing teeth

**Total
take-over**

√ in case of aspiration of a foreign body, or solid
food, remove it in the following manner:

. keep the nose closed so that the mouth opens and
give a few short taps on the uppermost part of his
back with the flat of the hand. If he does not cough
and expel the object immediately, perform the
Heimlich maneuver as described below

. if the patient turns blue after choking, apply
Heimlich's maneuver without delay: standing behind
the seated patient, put your arms round his waist.
With one hand make a fist with the thumb inside
and place the other hand round it. Place the fist
between the curve of the ribs and the navel and with
the other open hand powerfully thrust the fist
inward and upward in the abdomen. If necessary
repeat the thrusts several times. Through the
thrusting movement the air is explosively released
from the lungs and the foreign body is consequently
dislodged from the windpipe

. variation of Heimlich's maneuver for the supine
patient: place the left hand, clenched in a fist, on the
patient's stomach at the bottom of the sternum. Put
the right hand palm on the left fist, with the wrist
stretched at about 45 degrees. Subsequently thrust
the left hand downwards into the stomach with the
right hand in a jerking movement and press in the
direction of the sternum. Repeat this movement until
the foreign body has been dislodged and the patient
starts breathing again

√ always feed the patient in the sitting position

What the patient can do himself

as long as he is still able to move his head when sitting with his loins supported, he can, provided he is daily stimulated and passively exercised, spontaneously but not on command:

√ shriek if he experiences discomfort, such as caused by hunger, thirst, pain or a dirty incontinence system

√ slowly lift or turn his head for a short time

√ make grasping movements with his hands

√ clasp an object for a short time, if the palm of his hand comes into contact with it

√ from a spoon nip puréed food and swallow it slowly without chewing

√ slowly swallow liquids and semi-liquid or puréed food

√ push puréed food out of his mouth with his tongue

√ when being spoon fed, react to being touched on the corners of the mouth or the skin round the mouth by briefly opening his mouth and sometimes turning his head towards the spoon

√ he may still be able to cough when he aspirates food or liquids, but the cough reflex is weak and less efficient

Intervene observe for, and if necessary prevent

√ the necessity of placement of a feeding tube (i.e., a nasogastric tube or a gastrostomy). Disadvantages of a permanent tube in the stomach for forced feeding are:

- chewing, sucking, tongue and swallowing movements soon disappear and the mouth often remains open

- as a result of this there is a considerable decrease in the production of saliva, resulting in the oral cavity, tongue and lips becoming exsiccated, with infections (such as candida) of the mouth, tongue, pharynx and the lips soon occurring

- the patient becomes more isolated. The essential contact between the patient and his caregiver becomes restricted to a minimum

- increased predisposition to aspiration because of interference with the sphincter mechanisms, whereby regurgitation of stomach contents may occur. This happens in particular when the patient is in the supine position

√ spoon feeding or bottle feeding should always be done with the patient in the sitting position

Attitude   √ realize that the insertion of a permanent tube in the patient's stomach for forced feeding has significant consequences for his quality of life and the peace of mind of his family. The decision whether or not to insert the feeding tube should be taken by the medical and nursing team as a whole (multidisciplinary), and always in consultation with the relatives. Sometimes, medical conditions may require temporary placement of a feeding tube. Whenever placement of a permanent feeding tube is being considered, it should always be preceded by careful observation of the patient during meals for a longer period of time and a thorough medical examination. Through the exchange of information and the ensuing discussion, the team arrive at a clear formulation of the problem and of the consequences of a permanent tube placement. Only then is it possible to take a responsible decision. Inserting a permanent tube in the stomach must always be done with the interest of the patient in mind and not because it saves the caregiver time or because it is the easiest solution. It should never be a routine procedure.

What the patient can do himself

if he is no longer able to lift his head up on his own in the sitting or supine position, he still can, provided he is stimulated and passively exercised, for an indefinite time spontaneously:

√ react to loud sounds by blinking his eyes, heaving a deep sigh and sometimes by catching his breath

√ shriek and breathe rapidly and with flushing of his face when he has feelings of discomfort, such as caused by hunger, thirst, pain or a dirty incontinence system

√ clasp a finger around a finger or an object which comes into contact with the palm of the hand

√ if he is gently touched on the cheek, slowly direct his head to the side of the caressed cheek

√ make searching and sucking movements with his lips if the corners of his mouth or the skin round the mouth are touched

√ automatically start sucking when a stimulus, such as the nipple of a bottle is put in his mouth

√ swallow liquid or semi-liquid food very slowly in seated position

√ move his mouth to a stimulus, such as the nipple of a feeding bottle and grip it with his lips

√ refuse too much food or drink by passively allowing it to run out of his mouth

√ produce a faint inefficient cough when aspirating

Intervene observe for, and if necessary prevent

√ for the severly demented person, being nourished via a bottle with a nipple is a good alternative to feeding via a tube in the stomach. If the mouth or its surroundings are touched, the mouth instinctively opens and reflex sucking occurs. This makes it often possible to maintain the feeding process through the natural way

√ advantages of feeding through the mouth, as opposed to a feeding tube, are:
- the salivary glands and the swallowing reflexes continue to function
- eating may still cause a pleasurable sensation
- regular direct contact with the caregiver is maintained
- while eating, the patient moves his jaws, head, neck, shoulders, arms, hands and fingers

Partial take-over

√ bring the drinking bottle within the patient's field of vision until the nipple touches the corners of the mouth or the lips; reflex sucking movements are then set in motion when his lips clasp the nipple. If the food in the bottle is immediately attainable, the mouth sucks it up in short draughts. In this way the patient can to some extent regulate the tempo of the food intake

Total take-over

√ consult the dietician about the composition of the bottle feed: this must comprise all the necessary nutritional elements

√ keep his nose clean and instill decongesting drops if the nose is choked on account of a cold, in order to promote good respiration through the nose during the intake of food (avoid use of oily nose drops which, when passing into the lungs, may cause a chemical pneumonitis)

√ the patient should always be in the sitting position when being spoon fed or bottle fed

√ if the patient is no longer capable of drinking enough, or when the mouth is dry, moisten the mouth and lips and give him water with the aid of a gauze: put part of an ice cube in the middle of the gauze, bind the gauze round it and put this in the patient's mouth; hold onto the gauze. The ice block slowly melts in the mouth, has a cooling effect, quenches the thirst and promotes sucking and swallowing

Attitude

√ realize that feeding via the bottle, when it is no longer possible to feed via a spoon or drinking cup, is preferable to mechanical, impersonal and unnatural tube feeding via nasogastric tube or gastrostomy. The swallowing reflex and the tongue movements are usually intact but slow

What the patient can do himself	√ as long as he can still walk independently, he can still go to the toilet as described in stage IIIB for about one year
Total take-over	√ see stage III B **going to the toilet**
	√ as long as he can still walk independently, it is possible, provided he does not exhibit anxiety or resistance, to put him on the toilet or commode at regular intervals. While he is sitting, supervise him, reassure him and divert him, for example by singing, talking to him or stroking his back. He can no longer perform any purposeful action whatsoever
Attitude	√ realize that a dirty incontinence system causes considerable discomfort to the patient. Although it is often impossible to keep him dry all the time, changing the incontinence system before each meal and before he goes to bed greatly reduces distress. Restlessness at night can be caused by a dirty incontinence system

CHAPTER 6

THE LIMIT TEST

Explanation

The LIMIT test is intended as an aid to judging the functionality of the person who needs the help of a caregiver. As a result of the progression of the illness the patient with Alzheimer's disease finds it increasingly difficult to perform the routine activities involved in the care of the household and of his own body. In order to provide the most efficient and most effective help the caregiver must repeatedly be able to assess the extent to which the patient is still able to carry out these activities. The caregiver can determine this in two ways.

Firstly by examining the degree of insight the patient still has into the how and why of these activities and secondly by observing him or her in the performance of the activities.

The LIMIT test provides the caregiver with assessment criteria. Firstly by means of purposeful questions that assess the patient's practical knowledge as regards routine activities and secondly by means of letting him perform specific tasks with which the various component parts of the patient's self-care activities can be examined. Every complex activity calls for the ability to *oversee* it, the *preparation* or plan of action, the *accomplishment* of the plan and the *appraisal* of the desirability and of the result of the activity. These four components are successively tested for each of the four daily routine self-care activities: personal hygiene; dressing and undressing; eating and drinking; going to the toilet.

The questions are aimed at establishing what the patient knows about these activities; the tasks are aimed at assessing the patient's ability to perform the component parts of the activities in the concrete situation; his ability to operationalize his knowledge.

The everyday objects needed for the test are to be found in every house, rest home or nursing home and can if necessary be brought by the person doing the test.

Each question or group of questions and each task must be completed by the patient within the set time. This time limit is given for each question and task. By adding up the number of minutes within which the questions and tasks for a particular activity have to be completed, it is possible to calculate the time needed to test this specific activity. The total test takes two and a half hours. It can if necessary be done in a morning or an afternoon. However, it is not necessarily the intention that the test should take place all at one time. This does not usually lead to the best results. Patients with Alzheimer's disease frequently suffer from fear of failure. They are often suspicious and defensive. They feel ashamed if there are certain things they do not know and do everything possible to conceal this from other people and from themselves. Every patient uses his own individual strategy: some people make the excuse that they are too tired or not feeling well, others try to divert the person giving the test by steering the conversation to another topic, or they get upset and walk out, thus making it impossible to carry out the test.

In order to have the greatest possible chance of a successful test, a number of general conditions must be complied with:

1. The person who gives the test, hereafter called the caregiver/tester, must make sure that all the objects needed for the test are ready on a table or are present in the room, such as a fitted lavatory basin with faucets and a plug for the wastepipe.
   Having to look for objects distracts the patient. The time needed for the preparation of a particular test, for example walking to the lavatory basin, is not included in the set time. Only the time needed to answer the questions or perform the actual action is noted.

2. The test should ideally take place in a comfortable, but not too large room, where the patient and the caregiver can sit at a table together, quietly and informally, without being disturbed by third parties or by the telephone.

3. The patient often finds it pleasant to be asked to help the caregiver. Most of the questions and tasks have been drawn up in such a way that the caregiver can present them as a personal problem, for which he calls on the patient for advice. In this way the patient has the feeling that he is in control of the situation.

4. It is to be recommended that the caregiver takes as few notes as possible during the actual test and restricts himself to keeping the score.

The Score

1. The score for the answers to the questions and the results of the tasks is entered by encircling the figure 1 or the figure 0 in the appropriate column.
2. The figure 1 is encircled if a question has been correctly answered or a task properly performed within the allowed time period.
3. For an incorrect answer or no answer and a wrongly performed or not performed task within the allowed time period the figure 0 is encircled.
4. The correct answers are given in the 'criteria' column. For most of the questions several possible answers are given. The patient need only give one correct answer to score a point. For some questions there is only one correct answer. This is explicitly stated.
5. The tasks test the patient's ability to carry out certain actions with the aid of objects in general use with which everyone is familiar.
6. Under 'preparation of test' the preparations are listed which the caregiver has to carry out before giving the test.

The Test Scores

The test scores can be analysed from two angles:

1. In the first place with regard to the four activities of self-care: personal hygiene; dressing and undressing; eating and drinking; going to the toilet. This enables the caregiver/tester to gain insight into the nature of the specific activity, or the part thereof, with which the patient needs help.
2. In the second place the scores can be scrutinized from the point of view of the four components which constitute each activity: surveying, preparing, accomplishing and appraising the result of the activity.

By assessing the performance of the patient on each of the four constituent parts of a compound activity (such as for instance dressing), his inability to carry out that activity can now be analyzed. This analysis makes it possible to expose the strong and the weak points in the self-care of each individual patient.

With the aid of this information the caregiver can draw up a better plan for more specifically oriented help. This should ultimately lighten the caregiver's task, because it gives the patient more control and consequently may lessen his resistance.

Personal Hygiene

Surveying			Preparing			Accomplishing			Appraising		
task	no. of questions	no. correct	task	no. of questions	no. correct	task	no. of questions	no. correct	task	no. of questions	no. correct
1	15	....	18	1	....	22	19	....	24	1	....
2	3	....	19	1	....	23	16	....	25	1	....
3	1	....	20	1	....				26	1	....
4	1	....	21	1	....				27	1	....
5	1	....							28	1	....
6	2	....							29	1	....
7	1	....							30	1	....
8	1	....							31	1	....
9	1	....							32	13	....
10	1	....							33	4	....
11	1	....									
12	1	....									
13	3	....									
14	1	....									
15	30	....									
16	13	....									
17	70	....									

Dressing & Undressing

Surveying			Preparing			Accomplishing			Appraising		
task	no. of questions	no. correct	task	no. of questions	no. correct	task	no. of questions	no. correct	task	no. of questions	no. correct
34	4	....	50	4	....	51	8	....	57	6	....
35	3	....				52	1	....	58	4	....
36	4	....				53	14	....	59	1	....
37	1	....				54	1	....	60	1	....
38	1	....				55	2	....	61	1	....
39	3	....				56	2	....	62	1	....
40	2	....							63	1	....
41	1	....							64	1	....
42	4	....							65	1	....
43	4	....							66	4	....
44	4	....							67	1	....
45	3	....							68	1	....
46	1	....							69	3	....
47	1	....									
48	1	....									
49	32	....									

Eating & Drinking

Surveying			**Preparing**			**Accomplishing**			**Appraising**		
task	*no. of questions*	*no. correct*	*task*	*no. of questions*	*no. correct*	*task*	*no. of questions*	*no. correct*	*task*	*no. of questions*	*no. correct*
70	1	....	86	1	....	91	8	....	98	1	....
71	5	....	87	4	....	92	1	....	99	1	....
72	1	....	88	5	....	93	1	....	100	1	....
73	2	....	89	1	....	94	3	....	101	1	....
74	3	....	90	1	....	95	1	....	102	1	....
75	6	....				96	2	....	103	1	....
76	23	....				97	3	....	104	1	....
77	3	....							105	1	....
78	2	....							106	1	....
79	2	....							107	1	....
80	5	....							108	3	....
81	1	....							109	2	....
82	1	....							110	2	....
83	4	....							111	1	....
84	14	....							112	1	....
85	51	....							113	1	....
									114	5	....
									115	3	....

Going to the Toilet

Surveying			Preparing			Accomplishing			Appraising		
task	no. of questions	no. correct	task	no. of questions	no. correct	task	no. of questions	no. correct	task	no. of questions	no. correct
116	12	....	125	1	....	131	1	....	135	1	....
117	1	....	126	1	....	132	1	....	136	1	....
118	1	....	127	1	....	133	1	....	137	1	....
119	1	....	128	1	....	134	1	....	138	1	....
120	1	....	129	1	....				139	1	....
121	1	....	130	1	....				140	1	....
122	1	....							141	1	....
123	1	....							142	1	....
124	1	....							143	1	....
									144	1	....

Name of the patient: _____

Sex: ☐ male   ☐ female

Date of birth: _____

Country and   _____

   place of birth: _____

Education: _____

Resident: ☐ at home, no. of persons _____

                      ☐ rest home   ☐ nursing home

Primary caregiver   ☐ partner ☐ son ☐ daughter

                      ☐ non-professional ☐ professional

LIMIT stage: _____

Name of person giving test: _____

Date of test: _____

Survey of compound daily self-care activities	No. of questions	No. of tasks	Total time limit	Total no. correct answers
Personal Hygiene	33	210	60	_____
Dressing & Undressing	36	127	30	_____
Eating & Drinking	46	183	41	_____
Going to the Toilet	29	40	11	_____
Total LIMIT test	144	560	142	_____

Survey of constituent activities	No. of questions	No. of tasks	Total time limit	Total no. correct answers
Surveying	58	359	76	_____
Preparing	16	26	6	_____
Accomplishing	19	86	29	_____
Appraising	51	89	31	_____
Total LIMIT test	144	560	142	_____

	Personal hygiene		**Surveying**
Questions and Tasks	Right	Wrong or no answer	Criteria

Time limit 3 minutes

1. Name all parts of the body which have to be washed. Begin at the head.

(If necessary the caregiver encourages the patient with: "Yes, go on" or "Do you know any more parts of the body which have to be washed?"

Right	Wrong or no answer	Criteria
1	0	a. face
1	0	b. ears
1	0	c. neck
1	0	d. nape
1	0	e. arms
1	0	f. armpits
1	0	g. shoulders
1	0	h. hands
1	0	i. chest
1	0	j. stomach
1	0	k. genitals
1	0	l. legs
1	0	m. feet
1	0	n. back
1	0	o. bottom/buttocks/ anus

Time limit questions 2/14 is 5 minutes

2. What is the difference between:

	Right	Wrong or no answer	Criteria
a. deodorant & toothpaste?	1	0	*deodorant:* against body odor; you use it in your armpits *toothpaste:* to clean your teeth; you put it on a toothbrush
b. a shower & a bath?	1	0	*shower:* you stand; running water *bath:* you sit or lie; no running water

| Questions and Tasks | Personal hygiene | | Surveying |
	Right	Wrong or no answer	Criteria
c. a gas heater and an electric heater?	1	0	*gas heater:* is an appliance to heat water without gas *electric heater:* an appliance to heat water with electricity
3. Tell me, what is a pilot burner?	1	0	a small burner,eg in a stove, to keep it lighted
4. What is an electric outlet for?	1	0	to put in the plug of an electric appliance
5. Why is it dangerous to put the plug in the outlet with wet hands?	1	0	because you could get current through your body; because you could get a shock; because it could kill you

6. There are usually two faucets on a lavatory basin.

Questions and Tasks	Right	Wrong or no answer	Criteria
a. Why two faucets?	1	0	a. one for cold and one for hot water
b. Which faucet is the hot water faucet?	1	0	b. the left
7. What is a faucet for?	1	0	to draw water
8. How can I stop the water running away?	1	0	close off the wastepipe with a plug

	Personal hygiene		**Surveying**
Questions and Tasks	Right	Wrong or no answer	Criteria
9. What do you do if the bath (shower) is too cold?	1	0	adjust the faucet
10. What do you do if the toothpaste is finished (denture cleanser)?	1	0	buy new
11. Where can you buy toothpaste?	1	0	drugstore; supermarket
12. The doctor has given me a prescription, which says 1 tablet 3 times a day. Can you tell me what that means?	1	0	1 tablet in the morning, midday and evening

13. If I have to take 1 tablet 3 times a day, how many is that:

	Right	Wrong or no answer	Criteria
a. per day?	1	0	3 tablets
b. per week?	1	0	21 tablets
c. in the month of June?	1	0	90 tablets
14. Name 6 actions you perform when you wash your hands	1	0	a. turn on tap
	1	0	b. wet them
	1	0	c. soap them
	1	0	d. wash them
	1	0	e. rinse them
	1	0	f. dry them

Personal hygiene   Surveying

Time limit for question 15 A, B, C, is 8 minutes. The caregiver/tester lays out on the table the ten objects listed below, so that the patient can easily see them and point to them. The caregiver/tester sits close to the patient.

15A. (The caregiver/tester shows the objects one by one)
   'Tell me, what is this?'
15B. (The caregiver/tester names each object) and asks the patient:
   'Point to ....'
15C. (The caregiver/tester gives the patient the objects one by one) and asks:
   'What is this used for?'

	Quest.A right	Quest.A wrong	Quest.B right	Quest.B wrong	Quest.C right	Quest.C wrong	Criteria 15C
Objects							
1. nail scissors	1	0	1	0	1	0	cut nails
2. nail file	1	0	1	0	1	0	file nails
3. comb	1	0	1	0	1	0	comb hair
4. hairbrush	1	0	1	0	1	0	brush hair
5. washcloth	1	0	1	0	1	0	soap yourself
6. soap	1	0	1	0	1	0	clean yourself wash yourself
7. toothbrush	1	0	1	0	1	0	clean teeth
8. handkerchief or facial tissue	1	0	1	0	1	0	blow nose; wipe nose & mouth
9. electric shaver	1	0	1	0	1	0	remove hair, or shave
10. bath towel	1	0	1	0	1	0	dry body

	Personal hygiene		**Surveying**
Questions and Tasks	Right	Wrong or no answer	Criteria

Time limit question 16 is 5 minutes

16. 'Tell me, what can you do with your ...?'

a. nose	1	0	smell; blow; sniff; sneeze
b. ears	1	0	hear; listen
c. eyes	1	0	look; see; blink; wink
d. mouth	1	0	eat, talk; open and shut;
e. lips	1	0	give a kiss; grip; smack
f. tongue	1	0	taste; lick; talk; stick out
g. teeth	1	0	bite
h. molars	1	0	chew, grind food
i. arms	1	0	reach; wave; embrace
j. hands	1	0	work; take hold; caress; hit
k. fingers	1	0	grasp;hold;twiddle
l. legs	1	0	bend; walk;stand on
m. feet	1	0	stand on; walk; kick

Time limit question 17 is 8 minutes. The caregiver/tester sits at an arm's-length from the patient with no table between them.

Personal hygiene   Surveying

17A. (The caregiver/tester points to the 35 parts of the body, listed below, in himself)

'What do you call the part of the body I am pointing to?'

17B. (The caregiver/tester successively names the 35 parts of the body listed below)

'Point to the part of the body in yourself that I shall now name'

	17A		17 B			17A		17 B	
	r	w	r	w		r	w	r	w
Parts of the body					*Parts of the body*				
1. hair of the head	1	0	1	0	19. thumb	1	0	1	0
2. forehead	1	0	1	0	20. index finger	1	0	1	0
3. cheek	1	0	1	0	21. middle finger	1	0	1	0
4. right cheek	1	0	1	0	22. ring finger	1	0	1	0
5. ear	1	0	1	0	23. little finger	1	0	1	0
6. left ear	1	0	1	0	24. leg	1	0	1	0
7. mouth	1	0	1	0	25. left leg	1	0	1	0
8. lips	1	0	1	0	26. right leg	1	0	1	0
9. tongue	1	0	1	0	27. knee	1	0	1	0
10. teeth	1	0	1	0	28. calf	1	0	1	0
11. neck	1	0	1	0	29. ankle	1	0	1	0
12. shoulder	1	0	1	0	30. foot	1	0	1	0
13. armpit	1	0	1	0	31. big toe	1	0	1	0
14. arm	1	0	1	0	32. little toe	1	0	1	0
15. elbow	1	0	1	0	33. back	1	0	1	0
16. hand	1	0	1	0	34. stomach	1	0	1	0
17. left hand	1	0	1	0	35. buttocks	1	0	1	0
18. right hand	1	0	1	0					

	Personal hygiene		**Preparing**
Questions and Tasks	Right	Wrong or no answer	Criteria

Time limit for questions 18/21 is 2 minutes.

18. Name 2 things you need and which you put ready before you start to wash yourself.	1	0	hand towel, soap, shampoo
19. Name two measures to prevent slipping and falling during bathing & showering	1	0	have an anti-slip mat; sit on a chair; do not stand on one leg; hold on to hand grab; see floor is dry; ask for help (eg. getting into bath)
20. What is an anti-slip mat for?	1	0	to prevent slipping and falling
21. I am sitting in a bath filled with water. How can I prevent the bath emptying?	1	0	put the plug in the wastepipe

| Questions and Tasks | Personal hygiene | | Accomplishing |
	Right	Wrong or no answer	Criteria

Time limit questions 22 a/s is 10 minutes

22. (From question 22f onwards the caregiver/tester puts the objects into the patient's hand) 'I am going to give you some tasks. Show me how you. ...'

Questions and Tasks	Right	Wrong or no answer	Criteria
a. turn on this faucet?	1	0	turn on faucet
b. turn off this faucet?	1	0	turn off faucet
c. use these two faucets to mix hot and cold water, so that it is lukewarm?	1	0	mix hot and cold water
d. close off the wastepipe?	1	0	close the wastepipe
e. open the wastepipe of this lavatory basin?	1	0	open the plugged wastepipe
f. take the soap out of this box?	1	0	take soap out of wrapping
g. stick this bandaid on my hand?	1	0	stick bandaid on back of caregiver's hand
h. unscrew the cap of this tube of toothpaste?	1	0	unscrew cap
i. screw the cap on the tube of toothpaste	1	0	screw the cap on
j. switch on this blow-dryer (or shaver)? (caregiver puts plug into outlet)	1	0	get appliance going
k. cut a finger nail with these scissors?	1	0	make cutting movement round finger nail
l. comb your hair with this comb?	1	0	make combing movement over hair
m. dry your face with this bath towel?	1	0	make drying movement over face
n. clean your teeth with this toothbrush? (pretends to do it)	1	0	make brushing movement in mouth

| Questions and Tasks | **Personal hygiene** | | **Accomplishing** |
	Right	Wrong or no answer	Criteria
o. blow your nose with this tissue?	1	0	put tissue to nose and blow
p. take this cleansing tissue out of this box	1	0	pull a tissue out of the box
q. fill this glass with cold tap water? (Caregiver/tester goes to lavatory basin with patient & puts empty glass in his hand)	1	0	turn on tap, fill glass with cold water
r. take a sip of water and spit it out? (Caregiver/tester gives patient a glass with small amount of water)	1	0	spit the water out into the lavatory basin
s. put enough toothpaste on this brush to clean your teeth? (tube has already been opened)	1	0	put toothpaste onto hairs of the brush

Time limit for question 23 is 5 minutes.

Caregiver/tester and patient sit at arm's-length from one another without a table in between. With these tasks it is a question of whether the patient knows how the task has to be performed, not of whether he can do it entirely without hesitation.

23. 'I am going to ask you to do a number of things. Please do the things I ask.'

a. with your right index finger point to your left middle finger	1	0
b. put your left hand on your right thigh	1	0

| Questions and Tasks | Personal hygiene | | Accomplishing |
	Right	Wrong or no answer	Criteria
c. put your right hand round your neck	1	0	
d. hold your calves with both hands	1	0	
e. hold your right elbow with your left hand	1	0	
f. show me the palms of your hands	1	0	
g. raise two fingers	1	0	
h. raise eight fingers	1	0	
i. show me your teeth	1	0	if the patient has dentures, not correct if the dentures are taken out of the mouth
j. put your tongue out	1	0	
k. bend forward	1	0	
l. sit with your legs wide apart	1	0	
m. lift up your right leg	1	0	
n. point to your back	1	0	
o. turn your head to the right (do not strain the head)	1	0	look clearly to the right
p. put your left foot in my hand	1	0	

Personal hygiene			Appraising
Questions and Tasks	Right	Wrong or no answer	Criteria

Time limit for questions 24/31 is 5 minutes

Questions and Tasks	Right	Wrong or no answer	Criteria
24. Why is it important to wash yourself every day?	1	0	feel clean & fresh; be socially acceptable; otherwise you are smelly; prevent skin disorders; otherwise you may get vermin
25. My neighbor washes her whole body once a week. Why is that not enough?	1	0	see above
26. Mention two reasons why people are not able to wash themselves every day?	1	0	tired; ill; too much effort; pain; frightened of falling; forget
27. Why is it necessary to have ventilation in the bathroom/shower?	1	0	to remove steam; supply fresh air and remove stale air, to prevent giddiness
28. How can you tell whether the waste-pipe of the lavatory basin, bath or shower is blocked?	1	0	water does not run away (runs too slowly)
29. How can you see that a faucet is leaking?	1	0	faucet continues to drip after being turned off

	Personal hygiene		**Appraising**
Questions and Tasks	Right	Wrong or no answer	Criteria
30. How do you get a clogged waste-pipe unclogged?	1	0	use an unblocking agent; call plumber or relatives
31. Who do you see in the mirror? (Caregiver holds mirror in front of patient)	1	0	"that's me"; that is...(followed by own given name)

Time limit for question 32 a/m is 5 minutes.
(In between the questions the caregiver/tester answers 'now at least I know what to do')

32. 'Will you help me. What should I do if I:'

a. have a headache?	1	0	take an aspirin; put cold compress on forehead; call the doctor
b. notice that my feet hurt?	1	0	check for disorders of the feet; go to podiatrist or visit doctor; buy new shoes; put other pair of shoes on
c. have a grazed knee?	1	0	swab; put on a bandaid
d. have not had a bowel movement for four days?	1	0	adjust diet; buy a laxative; go to doctor
e. have a cold and a nasty cough?	1	0	buy medicine at drugstore; stay in bed; go to doctor
f. feel giddy?	1	0	sit/lie down; call doctor if it continues

	Personal hygiene		**Appraising**
g. think I have a fever?	1	0	take temperature; take an aspirin; stay in bed
h. have toothache for several days?	1	0	go to the dentist
i. pain with urinating?	1	0	go to the doctor; have urine examined
j. have a corn on my toe?	1	0	buy a corn plaster and put it on corn, see the podiatrist
k. have had a bad itch for a week?	1	0	go to the doctor
l. can hardly walk for pain in my knees?	1	0	go to physiotherapist, doctor; use a walking cane
m. have a running nose?	1	0	blow nose; use nose drops or anti-allergy remedy

Time limit of question 33 a/d is 4 minutes

33. Explain the meaning of this saying:

a. The eyes are the window of the soul	1	0	a person's eyes tell you a lot about his character
b. To have ones feet firmly on the ground	1	0	does not lose sight of reality
c. Give someone the cold shoulder	1	0	treat someone with contempt; refuse to talk to someone
d. The tongue is not steel, yet it cuts	1	0	slanderers hurt other people

Dressing & Undressing   Surveying

Questions and Tasks	Right	Wrong or no answer	Criteria

Time limit for questions 34/38 is 3 minutes.

34a (ask female patients). You are going to buy a skirt or dress. You want to buy a skirt or dress exactly like the one you have on (the patient now gives a description of the skirt or dress she has on). The shop assistant asks you the following questions:

a. What size do you take?	1	0	Caregiver estimates size of skirt or dress: - small=size 8-10 - medium=size 12-14 - large=size 16 and above
b. What color(s) do you want?	1	0	Caregiver judges color of skirt patient is wearing
c. What style of skirt (or dress) do you want: straight, pleated, flaired?	1	0	Caregiver judges style of skirt patient is wearing
d. Do you want the skirt length above or below the knee or ankle lenght?	1	0	Caregiver judges length of skirt patient is wearing

34b (ask male or female patients who wear pants). You are going to buy a pair of pants. You want to buy pants exactly like the pair you are wearing (the patient now gives a description of the trousers which he or she has on). The shop assistant asks the following questions:

a. What size do you take?	1	0	Caregiver judges the men's size in: -small=36-38-40 -medium=42 - 44 -large=46 & above see 34a for women's sizes

Dressing & Undressing Surveying

Questions and Tasks	Right	Wrong or no answer	Criteria
b. What color do you want?	1	0	
c. Do you want long pants or shorts?	1	0	
d. Do you want pants with or without turn-ups?	1	0	

35. (Give the patient pen and paper). The skirt (or trousers) costs $75.—
You pay with a hundred dollar bill.

a. how much change do you get	1	0	$25.—
b. write seventy five dollars in figures	1	0	$75.—
c. write $75.— in letters	1	0	seventy five dollars

36. You are also going to buy a pair of shoes. You want to buy shoes which look exactly like those you are wearing (the patient now gives a description of the shoes he or she has on).
The shop assistant asks the following questions:

a. What size shoes do you take?	1	0	Caregiver checks the shoe size
b. Do you want laced or step-in shoes?	1	0	Caregiver judges these features from the shoes the patient is wearing
c. With a leather or a rubber sole?	1	0	see b.
d. What color do you want?	1	0	see b.

37. You want to know how much money you have spent. The shoes cost $90.—, the skirt (or pants) costs $75.—. How much do these two items cost together?

	1	0	$165.—.

38. You had a total of $200.— with you. How much money have you got left?

	1	0	$35.—.

Dressing & Undressing   Surveying

Questions and Tasks	Right	Wrong or no answer	Criteria

The time limit for question 39-48 is 6 minutes.

39. Tell me what the difference is between:

a. sunglasses and reading glasses?	1	0	sunglasses: glasses with darkened lenses to protect the eyes against too bright sunshine (reading) glasses: aid to improve sight; 'for reading'; to be able to see better
b. a dress and a night-dress?	1	0	nightdress: garment worn at night in bed dress: outerwear for daytime
c. a suit & pajamas?	1	0	suit: daywear pajamas: nightwear

40. Name two garments which you put on:

a. if you are cold?	1	0	woolen sweater, scarf, winter coat waistcoat
b. if you are hot?	1	0	summer dress, thin blouse, summer pants, short-sleeved shirt, shorts
41. Name two ways of cleaning your own clothes	1	0	in the washing machine; at the laundry; hand wash

Dressing & Undressing   Surveying

Questions and Tasks	Right	Wrong or no answer	Criteria
42. When you start to dress yourself in the morning, which garment do you put on:			
a. first?	1	0	underwear: vest, undershirt, undershorts, panties/bra,slips
b. second (and after)?	1	0	see a.
c. third?	1	0	outerwear: blouse/ shirt, skirt/pants,dress
d. fourth?	1	0	see c.
43. (the caregiver/tester shows the patient one by one the objects listed below) I am going to show you several things. What is the name of:			
a. this object?	1	0	coat hanger
b. and of this?	1	0	mirror
c. and of this?	1	0	umbrella
d. and this?	1	0	clothespin
44. (next the caregiver/tester shows and names the objects) Tell me what this .... is used for.			
a. coat hanger	1	0	to hang up (without creasing) coat,dress blouse
b. mirror	1	0	to see myself in
c. umbrella	1	0	for protection against rain or sun
d. clothespin	1	0	to peg washing on a washing line
45. (the caregiver/tester puts a V-neck sweater in front of the patient). I have put a sweater in front of you. Show me:			
a. the inside of this sweater	1	0	
b. the front of this sweater	1	0	
c. the bottom	1	0	

Dressing & Undressing   Surveying

Questions and Tasks	Right	Wrong or no answer	Criteria

46. (the patient's coat is hanging on the coatrack amongst several other coats, the caregiver/tester accompanies the patient to the coatrack) Show me your coat.

    1   0

47. (the caregiver/tester puts a left, flat-heeled shoe on the table in front of the patient) On which foot does this shoe belong?

    1   0   the patient says 'the left foot' or points to left foot

48. (the caregiver/tester shows the sole of the shoe) Why is the sole of a shoe flat?

    1   0   gives stable balance; otherwise you may fall, wobble

Time limit for question 49 is 3 minutes. The caregiver/tester places the 16 objects named below, one by one, in a clearly recognizable form in front of the patient. The caregiver sits close to the patient.

Question 49A. 'Tell me, what is this?'
Question 49B. (The caregiver/tester names each object and garment) 'Show me .....'

	Quest.A Right Wrong		Quest.B. Right Wrong		Criteria
Objects					
1. wristwatch	1	0	1	0	(wrist)watch; clock
2. wedding ring	1	0	1	0	(wedding) ring
3. belt with buckle	1	0	1	0	belt, girdle
4. handkerchief	1	0	1	0	handkerchief
5. necktie	1	0	1	0	necktie
6. panties	1	0	1	0	panties; stockings

Dressing & Undressing   Surveying

Questions and Tasks

	Quest.A		Quest.B.		Criteria
	Right	Wrong	Right	Wrong	
Objects					
7. socks	1	0	1.	0	socks
8. flat shoe	1	0	1	0	shoe
9. bra	1	0	1	0	bra
10. underpants/ panties	1	0	1	0	underpants/ panties
11. shirt	1	0	1	0	shirt
12. blouse	1	0	1	0	blouse
13. sweater	1	0	1	0	sweater
14. trousers	1	0	1	0	trousers,pants
15. skirt	1	0	1	0	skirt
16. dress	1	0	1	0	dress

Dressing & Undressing   Preparing

Questions and Tasks	Right	Wrong or no answer	Criteria

Time limit for question 50 is 1 minutes. The caregiver/tester puts the following items of women's wear in front of the female patient: bra, panties, vest, blouse, skirt. For the male patient: trunks, vest, shirt, pants.

50. In front of you there are some articles of clothing. Which of these garments would you put on:

		Right	Wrong	Criteria
a.	first?	1	0	vest; panties; bra
b	second (& afterwards)?	1	0	see a.
c.	third? pants or skirt	1	0	blouse, shirt,
d.	fourth	1	0	see c. Note: both naming or pointing at the garment without naming it, is allowed

Dressing & Undressing   Accomplishing

Questions and Tasks	Right	Wrong or no answer	Criteria

51. I am going to give you several tasks. Please do what I ask:

a. (the caregiver/tester hands the patient a sturdy (wooden) coat hanger and a blazer/jacket). *Hang this jacket on this coat hanger.*

      1   0

b. (the caregiver puts 3 pairs of socks, of different colors, in front of the patient without sorting them). *Sort the socks into pairs.*

      1   0

c. (the caregiver puts an unfolded men's handkerchief in front of the patient). *Fold this handkerchief up in four*

      1   0

d. (the caregiver puts 6 folded men's handkerchiefs in front of the patient) *Put these handkerchiefs in a pile*

      1   0

e. (the caregiver puts a pair of shoes on the table with the toes towards the patient). *Put the right shoe next to the left, so that you can put them on*

      1   0

f. (the caregiver puts a flat-heeled shoe with a lace in front of the patient and gives him an easy to thread shoe lace).
    Thread this lace in this shoe

      1   0

g. (the caregiver puts a pair of folded sunglasses in front of the patient). *Put these sunglasses on*

      1   0

h. (the caregiver puts a matching eye glasses cover in front of the patient).
    Take the glasses off again and put them in this cover

      1   0

52. (The caregiver/tester hands over his own coat). *Please help me into this coat*

      1   0

The time limit for questions 53/57 is 4 minutes. The caregiver/tester lays out the following objects: garments with hooks and eyes; with buckle; with velcro; with snap fasteners; with zipper; with button and buttonhole; shoe with lace.

Dressing & Undressing   Accomplishing

Questions and Tasks	Right	Wrong or no answer	Criteria
53. Show me how you:			
a. open this hook & eye fastening	1	0	
b. close hook & eye fastening	1	0	
c. open this buckle (clasp with separate pivot and metal prong)			
	1	0	
d. fasten this buckle	1	0	
e. open this velcro fastening	1	0	
f. close this velcro fastening	1	0	
g. open this snap fastener	1	0	
h. close snap fastener	1	0	
i. open this zipper	1	0	
j. close this zipper	1	0	
k. open this button & buttonhole fastening	1	0	
l. close this button & buttonhole fastening	1	0	
m. undo this shoelace	1	0	
n. tie this shoelace	1	0	

54. (Give the patient a belt and a pair of pants with 6 loops)
Please thread this belt through the loops of these pants

                         1   0

55. (Let the patient put on a waistcoat, blazer or jacket with three buttons and help him if necessary with putting it on)

	Right	Wrong or no answer	Criteria
a. Let me see how you do up these buttons	1	0	do up the three buttons in the right holes
b. Undo the three buttons again	1	0	undo the buttons

Dressing & Undressing — Accomplishing

Questions and Tasks	Right	Wrong or no answer	Criteria
56. (Give the patient a scarf)			
a. Show me how you put this scarf on	1	0	put scarf round neck
b. Take the scarf off	1	0	take scarf off

Time limit for question 57 is 2 minutes

Questions and Tasks	Right	Wrong or no answer	Criteria
57. Tell me what you do if there is:			
a. a grease spot on your skirt (pants)	1	0	take to dry cleaner wash; use stain remover
b. a tear in your panties/ trunks	1	0	repair; throw away
c. a hole in your panties (sock) others; buy new	1	0	throw away; darn, repair sock; put on
d. a button is missing from your blouse (shirt)	1	0	sew on another button; put on another blouse (shirt)
e. a broken zipper	1	0	put in a new one or get dressmaker or cleaner to do it
f. trodden-down heels on your shoes	1	0	take to the shoemaker

Dressing & Undressing   Appraising

Questions and Tasks	Right	Wrong or no answer	Criteria

The time limit for questions 58/69 is 7 minutes.

58. Which season is it when:

	Right	Wrong or no answer	Criteria
a. it freezes and the trees are bare?	1	0	winter
b. it is warm and people lie on the beach in bathing suits?	1	0	summer
c. the leaves appear again on the trees?	1	0	spring
d. the leaves turn color and fall from the trees?	1	0	autumn; fall

59. It is raining and you get up to go shopping. What do you use to protect your clothing against the rain?

	Right	Wrong or no answer	Criteria
	1	0	raincoat, umbrella

60. (Give the patient a sock with a big hole in the toe). What is wrong with this sock?

	Right	Wrong or no answer	Criteria
	1	0	it has a hole in it

61. What do you do if there is a hole (or a ladder) in your sock/panties?

	Right	Wrong or no answer	Criteria
	1	0	throw it away; darn it if possible

62. Give one reason for regularly putting on clean panties/socks?

	Right	Wrong or no answer	Criteria
	1	0	spots between the toes; itching; socks (etc.) get smelly, dirty

Dressing & Undressing   Appraising

Questions and Tasks	Right	Wrong or no answer	Criteria
63. Give one reason why people buy a new pair of shoes	1	0	old ones were un-comfortable, pain-ful; lost their shape worn out; want something different
64. (The caregiver/tester shows the sole of a shoe with a hole in it) Why does this shoe need repairing?	1	0	there is a hole in it
65. Name two ways of checking if you have your clothes on properly after dressing	1	0	look at the garment feel it with your hands; look in the mirror; ask someone if it looks alright

66. (These tasks should be done without the aid of a mirror)
Show how, without a mirror, you check whether your:

	Right	Wrong or no answer	Criteria
a. pants, skirt or dress is done up	1	0	looks at fastenings and uses hand to check
b. blouse or shirt is hanging out of your trousers or skirt	1	0	uses hand to check the clothes round the waist
c. sleeve is twisted	1	0	looks at the sleeve and brings hand to arm
d. buttons are done up in the right order	1	0	looks at and feels the place where the buttons are attached

Dressing & Undressing   Appraising

Questions and Tasks	Right	Wrong or no answer	Criteria
67. Why do people look in the mirror during and after dressing?	1	0	to check whether their clothes are on properly
68. Why is it not necessary to look in the mirror when you are *un*dressing?	1	0	you do not have to check anything
69. Explain the meaning of this saying:			
a. Apparel makes the man	1	0	people often judge too much from out-ward appearances
b. Near is my shirt, but nearer is my skin	1	0	Everyone thinks of himself first
c. If the cap fits, wear it	1	0	Whoever feels guilty, can apply the allusion to himself

Eating & Drinking   Surveying

Questions and Tasks	Right	Wrong or no answer	Criteria

Time limit for questions 70/75 is 4 minutes.

70. Where, in which room in the house, is the cooker?	1	0	kitchen

71. Name:

a. 3 sorts of fresh vegetables	1	0	e.g, spinach, salad, string beans
b. 2 sorts of meat for the hot meal	1	0	e.g., steak, liver, chicken
c. 2 sorts of fresh fish	1	0	e.g., cod, sole, porgy, prawns
d. 1 sort of pulse	1	0	e.g., dried brown beans, chick-peas, lentils
e. 3 sorts of fresh fruit	1	0	e.g., apples, straw-berries, melon, oranges

72. Vegetables and fruit can be bought fresh, but also in other forms. Name 2 other forms	1	0	(deep) frozen; canned; dried

73. Can you tell me the difference between:

a. boiled & fried potatoes	1	0	boiled in water; fried in pan with cooking fat or oil
b. mashed potatoes and french fries	1	0	boiled and mashed; cut into strips & deep fried in fat or oil

Eating & Drinking   Surveying

Questions and Tasks	Right	Wrong or no answer	Criteria
74. Let's suppose we eat together this evening. How much of these items do you think we need for 2 people?			
a. string beans	1	0	1 to 1/2 pound; two handfuls
b. potatoes	1	0	2 to 4
c. steak	1	0	1/2 to 3/4 of a pound
75. Can you tell me where I can buy ... ?			
a. fresh string beans	1	0	grocer/ supermarket
b. steak	1	0	butcher/supermarket
c. fresh fish	1	0	fishmonger/super-market
d. fresh fruit	1	0	grocer/ supermarket
e. pot of preserves	1	0	grocer/supermarket
f. dishtowel	1	0	department store/ supermarket

Supermarket counts as a right answer, provided the right department is given in answer to further questioning.

Time limit for question 76a/w is 6 minutes. Test requirements:
Copy out the sums so that the text is enlarged. Put the sums in front of the patient one by one, or cover up the text so that only one sum is visible at a time. The caregiver/tester reads the sum aloud while the patient reads with him. The caregiver scores the patient's answer.
The object of this section of the test is to see whether the patient can make the calculation, not whether he can read or write.

76.

	Right	Wrong or no answer	Criteria
a. 1 package of coffee costs $2.50. How much do I have over from $10.- if I buy 3 packages?	1	0	$2.50

Eating & Drinking   Surveying

Questions and Tasks	Right	Wrong or no answer	Criteria
b. Peter has 2 brothers & 3 sisters. Mother gives her children 20 cherries each. How many cherries does mother give altogether?	1	0	120 cherries
c. 5 people divide out 45 plums. How many plums have they altogether?	1	0	45 plums
d. A lady buys a table-cloth for a table 6 feet long by 2 feet wide. How old is she?	1	0	"You're tricking me"; you cannot find out from this question
e. Mary eats 3 times a day. How many times does she eat per week?	1	0	21 times
f. If Mary eats 3 times a day, how many times does she eat in the month of September?	1	0	90 times
g. 6 people are sitting at table. On the table is a plate with 18 slices of cheese. If the cheese is divided out exactly, how many slices of cheese does each person get?	1	0	3 slices of cheese
h. At the check-out you have to pay $45.-. You hand over a hundred dollar bill. How much change do you get?	1	0	$55.-
i. You have $25. - in your purse. You buy 1 package of coffee for $2.50	1	0	I have money over

	Eating & Drinking			**Surveying**
Questions and Tasks	Right	Wrong or no answer	Criteria	

		Right	Wrong or no answer	Criteria
	1 loaf of bread for $2.00 1 pound of cheese for $3.50 Will you be short of money or have money over?			
j.	There are 30 tea bags in a package. You need 2 bags to make a pot of tea. How many times can you make a pot of tea?	1	0	15 times
k.	You need one quart of milk. You buy a half gallon pack. How much milk do you have over?	1	0	one quart
l.	There are 12 fish sticks in a deep- freeze pack. For 3 people you fry 2 each. How many fish sticks do you have over?	1	0	6 fish sticks
m.	You buy 7 apples. You eat one apple a day. How many days can you eat an apple?	1	0	7 days; one week
n.	Spinach costs $1.50 per pound. How much do 2 pounds cost?	1	0	$3.-.
o.	Potatoes cost $0.80 per pound. How much does 1/2 pound cost?	1	0	$0.40
p.	Pears cost $1.20 per pound. What does 1/2 pound cost?	1	0	$0.60
q.	What do the products from questions n,o,p cost together?	1	0	$4.—

Eating & Drinking   Surveying

Questions and Tasks	Right	Wrong or no answer	Criteria
r. Steak costs $3.50 per half pound. How much does a pound cost?	1	0	$7.—
s. Ground meat costs $4.— per pound. What does 1 1/2 pound cost?	1	0	$6.—
t. Cheese costs $6.— per pound. What does 1/3 of a pound cost?	1	0	$2.—
u. What do the products from questions r,s,t cost altogether?	1	0	$15.—
v. What is the total cost of all the shopping (n/t)	1	0	$19.—
w. You pay with a twenty dollar bill. How many quarters do you get back?	1	0	4 quarters

Time limit for question 77 a,b and c is 3 minutes. Copy the clocks so that they are enlarged. Put the clocks in front of the patient one by one or cover the clocks up so that the patient only sees one at a time.
The caregiver/tester reads the task aloud, while the patient reads with him. The patient draws the figures and the hands in the clock. If no clear distinction is to be seen between the big hand and the little hand, ask the patient to point to them. If he points to the right hands, he scores for the right answer.

77.

	Right	Wrong or no answer	Criteria
a. This is the dial of a clock. Put the 12 figures in for the hours	1	0	12 figures correctly placed

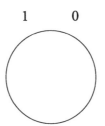

	Eating & Drinking		**Surveying**
Questions and Tasks	Right	Wrong or no answer	Criteria

	Right	Wrong or no answer	Criteria
b. Draw the big hand and little hand in the clock to show ten past nine	1	0	Small hand pointing to the nine, large hand pointing to the two
c. We eat at six o'clock. It takes three quarters of an hour to get the meal. Show me by drawing the hands of the clock what time I must start to prepare the meal.	1	0	Indicate quarter past five. Small hand points to five Big hand points to three.

Time limit questions 78/82 is 3 minutes.

78 (The caregiver/tester puts a set of metal tableware and a set of disposable plastic tableware in front of the patient)

	Right	Wrong or no answer	Criteria
a. What is the difference between this spoon, knife and fork?	1	0	metal is durable, plastic is thrown away after use; solid, not solid
b. Why is plastic tableware in use?	1	0	for convenience; no cleaning necessary

79. (The caregiver/tester shows a fork)

	Right	Wrong or no answer	Criteria
a. Name 2 sorts of food you do not eat with a fork	1	0	soup; yogurt
b. Why can you not eat soup with a fork?	1	0	it drips through the prongs of the fork

Eating & Drinking Surveying

Questions and Tasks	Right	Wrong or no answer	Criteria
80. (The caregiver/tester gives the patient a knife which clearly has a sharp and a blunt edge)			
a. Show me the sharp edge of this knife	1	0	
b. Show me the blunt edge of this knife	1	0	
c. What is the difference between the sharp and blunt edge of a knife?	1	0	you can cut with the sharp edge, not with the blunt edge
d. Name 2 actions you can do with a knife	1	0	cut;spread;push food on the fork;peel
e. Which is the cutting edge of this knife?	1	0	points to sharp edge
81. What happens if you put a pan of rice on to cook without enough water?	1	0	rice burns on
82. Why is it not desirable to swallow chewing gum?	1	0	it is not digested; it is not meant to be eaten, it is not food

Time limit questions 83-84 is 3 minutes

83.			
a. Which of the two, wine or detergent, can you drink?	1	0	wine
b. What do you use wine for?	1	0	to drink; to use in cooking;
c. What do you use detergent for?	1	0	to disinfect; to kill germs; to cleanse things

	Eating & Drinking		**Surveying**
Questions and Tasks	*Right*	*Wrong or no answer*	*Criteria*

		Right	Wrong or no answer	Criteria
d.	How do you know whether wine or detergent is in the bottle?	1	0	read the label; smell

84. (The caregiver/tester puts in front of the patient 5 identical wide, shallow bowls containing sugar, salt, pepper, mustard and ketchup. He must not name the contents as he puts the bowls down).

		Right	Wrong or no answer	Criteria
a.	How many bowls are there?	1	0	five
b.	These bowls contain sugar, salt, pepper, mustard and ketchup. Please give me:			
	the sugar	1	0	
	the salt	1	0	
	the pepper	1	0	
	the mustard	1	0	
	the ketchup	1	0	
c.	What is this?	1	0	the sugar
	What is this?	1	0	the salt
	What is this?	1	0	the pepper
	What is this?	1	0	the mustard
	What is this?	1	0	the ketchup

(if the patient answers 'I don't use that' for points d, e or f, ask him: 'what do people generally do in/on...?')

		Right	Wrong or no answer	Criteria
d.	What do you put in a cup of coffee: salt, sugar or pepper?	1	0	sugar
e.	What do you put on your boiled egg: sugar, salt or mustard?	1	0	salt
f.	What do you put on a frankfurter?	1	0	mustard

Eating & Drinking   Surveying

Time limit for question 85 A, B and C is 10 minutes.
The caregiver/tester lays the 17 objects, listed below, out on a table so that they are clearly visible to the patient, who can easily see them and point to them.

85
a. (Caregiver shows objects one by one) 'Tell me, what is this?'
b. (Caregiver names each object) 'Show me or point to the....'
c. (Caregiver gives the patient the objects one by one) 'Tell me what you use this for?'

Objects	Quest. A right	Quest. A wrong	Quest. B right	Quest. B wrong	Quest. C right	Quest. C wrong	Criteria 85c
1. teaspoon	1	0	1	0	1	0	stir
2. tablespoon	1	0	1	0	1	0	eat, scoop
3. soup ladle	1	0	1	0	1	0	serve out soup
4. fork	1	0	1	0	1	0	spear or eat solid food
5. chopsticks	1	0	1	0	1	0	eat solid food
6. potato knife	1	0	1	0	1	0	peel
7. dinner knife	1	0	1	0	1	0	cut, spread
8. tumbler	1	0	1	0	1	0	drink
9. cup with handle	1	0	1	0	1	0	drink
10. drinking straw	1	0	1	0	1	0	suck up liquid
11. corkscrew	1	0	1	0	1	0	uncork bottle
12. can opener	1	0	1	0	1	0	open can
13. egg timer	1	0	1	0	1	0	set cooking time
14. frying pan	1	0	1	0	1	0	fry; sauté
15. saucepan	1	0	1	0	1	0	boil
16. box of matches	1	0	1	0	1	0	make something burn, ignite something
17. dish towel	1	0	1	0	1	0	wipe up washed up dishes

	Eating & Drinking			**Preparing**

Questions and Tasks	Right	Wrong or no answer	Criteria

Time limit for questions 86/90 is 2 minutes

86. (Caregiver/tester puts a shallow plate, a deep plate and a saucer in front of the patient) There are three plates in front of you. From which of the plates can you eat soup?   1   0   deep plate

87. (The patient answers a, b and c without visual aids. For a, b and c the patient must name all the items specified) Tell me what you need to:

a. make a cup of tea?	1	0	tea, a cup, boiling water
b. toast a slice of bread?	1	0	slice of bread, toaster with plug in outlet
c. make a bowl of instant soup?	1	0	pan, measuring cup, water, whisk &/or spoon, source of heat (gas or electric), pack soup
d. fry an egg?	1	0	an egg, frying pan, butter, fork or knife, source of heat

88. (Tester puts tableware listed below in front of the patient.) There is tableware on the table in front of you. With which of these objects do you:

a. eat soup?	1	0	tablespoon
b. spear a carrot?	1	0	fork
c. butter bread?	1	0	knife as used for the meal, knife with rounded edge
d. peel a potato?	1	0	knife with sharp point
e. eat Chinese food (rice, meat, chicken, vegetables)?	1	0	chopsticks or fork and knife

| Questions and Tasks | **Eating & Drinking** | | **Preparing** |
	Right	Wrong or no answer	Criteria
89. Why is it sensible not to fill a cup or glass up to the brim?	1	0	to avoid spilling
90. Why do people use a table napkin while eating?	1	0	to avoid getting food on their clothes

Questions and Tasks	Eating & Drinking		Accomplishing
	Right	Wrong or no answer	Criteria

Time limit for questions 91/97 is 5 minutes.

91. (Put an empty bottle with screw top, a canister with hinged lid, a closed 8 oz. pack of milk and a latchkey in front of the patient). Show me how you:

a. screw the top off the bottle?	1	0	
b. screw the top on the bottle again?	1	0	
c. open the cookie box?	1	0	
d. close the box again?	1	0	
e. open the pack?	1	0	
f. close the pack again?	1	0	
g. open the front door with your (this) key?	1	0	
h. close and lock the front door?	1	0	close door, put key in lock, turn and take out of lock

92. (Put a wax light in front of the patient and give him a box of matches). Take a match out of the box and light the candle

	1	0	take match out of box, strike, light candle & blow out match in time

93. (Place a socket and a cord with a plug in front of the patient). Put this plug into the socket   1   0

94. (Put on the table in front of the patient two cups and saucers, two teaspoons, a lightweight teapot, half filled with cold tea and a sugar pot. The patient pours out first, then the caregiver/tester pours out tea for himself. If the patient cannot perform task a, pouring out, tasks b and c can be carried out using the caregiver's cup. Tasks a, b and c to be given separately.)

| Questions and Tasks | **Eating & Drinking** | | **Accomplishing** |
	Right	Wrong or no answer	Criteria
Here is a teapot filled with tea.			
a. Please pour out a cup of tea for me	1	0	without spilling, not filled to the brim
b. Put two spoonfuls of sugar in the cup	1	0	without spilling
c. Stir up the sugar	1	0	stir without spilling

95. (Caregiver/tester accompanies patient to sink and gives him a half-filled glass of water) There is still some water in this glass. Please throw it away in the sink

	1	0	knows how to throw liquid away

96. (Caregiver/tester puts a shallow plate, soft butter in a butter dish and a metal dinner knife which cuts easily in front of the patient. Tasks a and b to be given separately)

a. Please spread this slice of bread with this butter for me	1	0	reasonable amount of butter smeared over slice of bread
b. Now cut the bread into four equal pieces	1	0	know how to cut slice of bread into pieces

97. (Caregiver/tester puts a shallow plate with knife and fork in front of the patient and gives him a banana). Here is a banana

a. Please peel the banana and put the banana on the plate	1	0	peel off rind, put banana on plate
b. Using the knife and fork cut the banana into pieces	1	0	cut with aid of knife and fork
c. Put a piece of banana on the fork and put it in your mouth	1	0	spear the banana and put in the mouth without letting it fall off the fork

	Eating & Drinking		**Appraising**
Questions and Tasks	Right	Wrong or no answer	Criteria

Time limit for questions 98/115 is 5 minutes.

98. Why does a dish towel have to be washed regularly?	1	0	it gets dirty; it gets smelly
99. How often must you clean the working surface of the drainboard?	1	0	once a day
100. Can you tell me what you need to clean dirty crockery and cutlery?	1	0	hot water with a detergent in it; dishwashing mop; dishwasher
101. What do you do with small bits of food left over on the plate?	1	0	throw away in the garbage can; rinse down the sink
102. Where do you keep food left over from the meal and which you do not want to throw away?	1	0	refrigerator
103. Why do people get flies, mice or cockroaches in the kitchen?	1	0	through not regularly cleaning cupboards containing unwrapped food or food wrapped in

paper; through not cleaning kitchen appliances and kitchen floor; leaving food left-overs uncovered on drainboard of the sink

Eating & Drinking   Appraising

Questions and Tasks	Right	Wrong or no answer	Criteria
104. Why must the refrigerator be cleaned regularly?	1	0	to prevent mold, stale air and tainted food
105. How does mold start in the refrigerator?	1	0	not properly cleaned or temperature too high; food in refrigerator not regularly inspected
106. When does the kitchen garbage can need emptying?	1	0	when it is full or when the contents stink
107. How do you know when meat, chicken or milk have gone off?	1	0	smells tainted; presence of mold; milk looks curdled, it is past the expiry date on the package

108. What does tainted .... look like?

	Right	Wrong or no answer	Criteria
a. bread	1	0	mold on it
b. fruit	1	0	rotting, dark spots
c. soup	1	0	has froth on it

109. (Caregiver/tester gives patient a glass of orange juice). I have poured you out something to drink. Can you tell me:

	Right	Wrong or no answer	Criteria
a. what is in the glass?	1	0	orange juice
b. whether this is a hot or a cold drink?	1	0	cold

110. Can you tell me what happens if you:

	Right	Wrong or no answer	Criteria
a. let food burn on?	1	0	smell of burning; smoke, smoke alarm goes off

Eating & Drinking   Appraising

Questions and Tasks	Right	Wrong or no answer	Criteria
b. pour boiling water over your hand?	1	0	skin burns; blisters on the skin
111. How can you prevent the pan catching fire when frying or deep-frying?	1	0	turn the heat down in time
112. How do you know when potatoes are done?	1	0	when the prongs of a fork easily go into the potato
113. How do you know when chicken is done?	1	0	no longer a rosy color, comes away from bone easily
114. Can you tell me why:			
a. you must not pull a plug out of an outlet with wet hands?	1	0	you can get an electric shock, it is dangerous
b. you must blow out a burning match as soon possible?	1	0	otherwise you burn your fingers; letting it fall because it is painful may cause a fire
c. when something is boiling on the cooker, the heat must be turned down?	1	0	to prevent it boiling over and too much steam forming
d. the gas or electric flame or burner of the cooker must be turned out after use?	1	0	you can burn your fingers on it; there can be a fire; the flame can blow out with the risk

	Eating & Drinking		**Appraising**
Questions and Tasks	*Right*	*Wrong or no answer*	*Criteria*
			of gas poisoning or an explosion
e. a hot pan must be taken hold of with pot holders?	1	0	to prevent burning your fingers
115. Explain the meaning of this saying:			
a. take something with a grain of salt	1	0	things are not taken too literally (too seriously)
b. he does not look as if butter would melt in his mouth	1	0	he will get what he is entitled to
c. eaten bread is soon forgotten	1	0	generosity/blessings are soon forgotten

Going to the toilet   Surveying

Questions and Tasks	Right	Wrong or no answer	Criteria

116. This task is intended to test the patient's spatial power of conception. The drawing must not be turned upside down. Copy the drawing and put it in front of the patient. The drawing shows a plan of a house. The assignment consists of eleven questions and one drawing task. Time limit for this is 3 minutes.

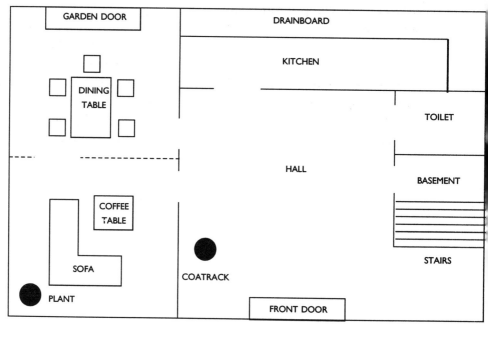

		Right	Wrong or no answer	Criteria
a.	you enter the house through the front door. If you stand with your back to the door, what do you see on your right?	1	0	the stairs
b.	behind the stairs you see two spaces, namely...	1	0	the toilet
c.	and the ...	1	0	the basement
d.	is the toilet on the left or right side?	1	0	right-hand side

Going to the toilet   Surveying

Questions and Tasks	Right	Wrong or no answer	Criteria
e. If you look sideways to the left in the hall, you see...	1	0	the coatrack
f. straight ahead at the end of the hall you see...	1	0	the kitchen
g. where there is a	1	0	drainboard
h. if you stand in the dining room with your back to the garden door, you look straight into the lounge. But there is a table in between. Which?	1	0	dining table
i. if you stand with your back to the draining board in the kitchen and face the front door, on which side is the coatrack?	1	0	right-hand side
j. and on which side is the toilet?	1	0	left
k. and on which side is the dining room?	1	0	right
l. you must go to the toilet and you are in the lounge by the plant. You want to get there as fast as possible by the shortest way. Draw the route you will take on the house plan.	1	0	the shortest way, without a détour. Patient draws a line from the plant to the toilet

Time limit questions 117/124 is 3 minutes.

117. We are together in a restaurant and you must go to the toilet. How do you find out where the toilet is?	1	0	look for the notice saying toilet, ladies, gentlemen; ask a waiter; ask your table companion to go with you.

Going to the toilet   Surveying

Questions and Tasks	Right	Wrong or no answer	Criteria
118. You want to go back to your table in the restaurant. How do you find your way back?	1	0	notice the way you went to the toilet; hope for the best; ask someone
119. Tell me, what is toilet paper for?	1	0	to clean up/wipe off (urine or feces)
120. What is a toilet brush for?	1	0	clean the inside of the toilet bowl
121. Why does a toilet bowl have a water flush?	1	0	to flush away (urine and feces)
122. About how many times a week does a person have a bowel movement?	1	0	4 to 7 times
123. In what part of the body do you have pain if your bowel movement was too hard or too runny?	1	0	in the stomach, in the belly
124. Why is it necessary to wash your hands after going to the toilet?	1	0	hygiene, prevent harmful bacteria being transmitted to yourself or other people, or to food or objects

Time limit for questions 125/130 is 1 minute

125. In a restaurant you enter the toilet & see that there is no toilet	1	0	take tissue out of your bag or pocket; look in another

Going to the toilet   Preparing

Questions and Tasks	Right	Wrong or no answer	Criteria
paper left. What do you do?			toilet for paper; wait until there is paper; ask the attendant
126. Why do you put the light on in a toilet without daylight?	1	0	to see what I am doing; otherwise I shall fall; otherwise I cannot see anything.
127. Why do adults close the door when they are in the toilet?	1	0	prevent spread of unpleasant smell; do not wish to be seen, privacy
128. Why do people not want anyone else present when they void or have a bowel movement?	1	0	shame; do not dare or cannot void or evacuate; some-else has no business to be there
129. How do you prevent your clothes getting soiled when you sit on the toilet bowl?	1	0	pull clothes far enough up or down and if necessary hold on to them
130. At times it can be difficult to reach the toilet on time. What can you use to to prevent your clothing getting wet when you have an accident?	1	0	incontinence system diaper; sanitary napkin

	Going to the toilet		**Accomplishing**
Questions and Tasks	Right	Wrong or no answer	Criteria

Time limit for questions 131/134 is 1 minute

131. You go to the toilet and want to open the door, but it is locked or there is the 'engaged' sign. What do you do?	1	0	wait; knock to see if anyone is there and wait; go away and return later
132. What do you do with the toilet paper you have used?	1	0	throw into the toilet bowl
133. Name 4 actions which must be performed directly after voiding and having a bowel movement.	1	0	take toilet paper; wipe clean; throw paper into toilet bowl;stand up; flush
134. You see that your urine (water) looks red. What do you do?	1	0	go to the doctor; mention it to someone in the family or to the person who helps you

Going to the toilet   **Appraising**

Questions and Tasks	Right	Wrong or no answer	Criteria

Time limit for questions 135/144 is 3 minutes

135. (Caregiver/tester shows written text 'ladies' and 'men')
When you go to a public toilet, you see the following indication. On one door there is this and on the other that. Which door do you go in?

    1   0   woman answers 'ladies'; man answers 'men'

136. Copy and enlarge the pictogram of man and woman. Caregiver/tester shows the enlarged pictogram to the patient.
You may also see this on the toilet door. Which door must you choose?

    1   0   woman points to female figure; man to male figure

137. Why are the toilet bowl and the toilet seat regularly cleaned?

    1   0   to prevent the transmission of bacteria

138. How do you know that the anus is clean after a movement?

    1   0   when there is no more feces on the toilet paper

139. What is the result of not or not properly wiping off the anus after a movement?

    1   0   dirty panties/under-pants; unpleasant smell

	Going to the toilet		Appraising
Questions and Tasks	Right	Wrong or no answer	Criteria
140. What do you do to be sure that your clothes are in order before you leave the toilet?	1	0	look at your clothes and feel with your hands; if possible look in the mirror
141. How does a person know that his move-ment is much too hard? (has trouble with constipation?)	1	0	when you have to press too hard, when it hurts
142. How does a person know that his movement is too thin?	1	0	the movement is watery
143. What are the symp-toms if a person complains of hemorrhoids?	1	0	tangible bulge in the anus, itching & sometimes pain
144. Explain the meaning of this saying: "I can feel it in my water/blood".	1	0	I know for sure

PREVENTING FALLS

Loss of equilibrium is one of the most frequently occurring problems of aging. With Alzheimer's disease, this disposition is augmented, and the chance of a fall increases as the illness progresses. Particularly in the later stages of the illness, the motor system, and especially the balance reflexes, become increasingly disturbed. Increased rigidity of the muscles with stiffening of the limbs, a flexed posture and small hesitant steps add to the risk. The visual impressions are often confounding and the patient's heightened urge to move makes the risk of falling even greater.

In the nursing home this increased risk of falling is frequently a reason for strapping these patients into their wheelchair or restchair as a precaution. As a consequence, the patient prematurely loses the ability to walk. Walking is usually the principal activity which still remains for the patient, particularly in the later stage of the disease. The caregiver who wants to keep the patient ambulatory for as long as possible, must be aware of all the situations which are accompanied by a higher risk of falling, so that he can take measures to make the patient's environment safer. He must continually gauge the patient's physical and mental condition.

A fall often leads to a fractured hip, shoulder, wrist, pelvis, skull or other part of the body, and this may be accompanied by serious soft tissue damage.

A fall on the head can give rise to a subdural hematoma: an accumulation of blood between the brain and the outermost and toughest of the three cerebral membranes which lie between the brain and the skull. This leads to compression of the underlying brain tissue. Some time after the fall, increasing confusion (delirium), general passivity and drowsiness occur and the patient gradually drifts into a coma. Not diagnosing a subdural hematoma in good time can lead to death. In the elderly, this condition can occur after a relatively minor head trauma.

A fracture results in pain and anxiety, lengthy medical and paramedical treatment, often permanent disability, and an increasing need of help and decreased socio-recreational opportunities.

Avoiding falls by taking general preventive measures

Every attempt should always be made to discover the cause of a fall. In particular if a patient is subject to falls. The caregiver should collect as much information as possible about the circumstances in which falling occurs and report it to the physician.

When does falling occur: during the day, in the evening, at night, during or after particular activities, during restless periods, does it happen often and how often? It is important to gather all the information possible. Many causes of falling can easily be prevented.

Causes of falls

1. *Causes related to the feet and legs:* swollen ankles and legs; ill fitting or too slippery shoes; wearing of bedroom slippers or mules instead of shoes; walking on stocking feet; loss of sensation in the feet and legs due to peripheral neuropathy (dysfunction of the nerves of the leg); vascular problems; too cold feet; arthritis. These factors all influence the pattern of walking and decrease stability.

2. *Giddiness and fainting (syncope)* resulting from: excessive straining on the toilet; excessive bending backwards of the head; weight loss and weakness because of poor eating; medicines such as diuretics, sedatives, tranquillizers and antihypertensives; hypotensive episodes; irregular heart action; sudden drop in blood pressure.
    It is important to encourage the patient to:
    - wait about fifteen minutes after a meal before walking about. In older people a drop in blood pressure often occurs during and after eating, resulting in giddiness and sometimes fainting.
    - remain seated while showering, bathing and dressing. The warm water can cause dilation of the blood vessels; the blood pressure drops, resulting in giddiness and sometimes fainting.

3. *Drowsiness,* resulting from: insufficient intake of fluid, alcohol, medicines such as sedatives and tranquillizers, or a febrile illness.

4. *Lack of sleep:* It is important to examine the cause of insufficient sleep and restlessness at night before prescribing sleeping pills which can lead to drowsiness, confusion and more difficulty in moving during the day, with resultant disturbances of the equilibrium when walking. Irritability and excitement can sometimes also follow the use of these medicaments in patients with dementia.

   Nocturia, the need to get up to urinate during the night, is one of the more frequent causes of sleep deprivation and of falls in elderly patients.

5. *Shortness of breath,* resulting from: maintaining too high a pace for the patient in the caregiving process, or shallow and rapid breathing because of fear, bad ventilation or emphysema.

6. *Tiredness* resulting from: increased urge to move; drinking too little; eating too little; certain medications

7. *Poor vision,* resulting from: not wearing ones glasses, dirty glasses; inadequate lighting during the day and at night; eye diseases such as glaucoma (too high pressure in the eyeball) or cataract.

   With aging, the keenness of light and color perception decreases. Adjusting to the dark becomes more difficult as a result of decreased vision in dim light.

   Clouded sight after the use of eye drops can also lead to falls: the patient should wait about twenty minutes before getting up and moving about. The patient does not always notice that his sight is clouded. Dark patches on the floor and on the street can be mistaken for holes, which the patient steps over with a big stride or tries to walk round. Because of an impaired sense of equilibrium many elderly patients depend more on their vision, and constantly keep their eyes on the floor or ground.

8. *Poor hearing,* resulting from: incorrectly tuned hearing aid, refusal to wear the hearing aid; accumulation of wax in the ears.

   Sounds may be heard, but not recognized or localized.

   Unexpected, loud noises and approaching the patient from behind should be avoided. Always warn the patient when assisting him, or he may startle and can lose his balance.

9. *Unsafe living conditions,* such as: a room with too many objects with too little space for the patient to move; loose or curled up rugs or mats on the floor; a loose stair carpet; slippery floors; loose leads; books or other objects on the floor; inadequate lighting; use of inadequate furniture such as too low chairs without armrests or a wobbly table; uneven

flagstones or tiles in the garden or on the balcony; wobbly or too low chairs; lack of a stool in the shower; lack of nonslip mats in the bathtub or shower; lack of, or failure to make use of handgrasps in the toilet and bathroom; lack of bed rails; too low room temperature

10. *Inadvertent actions of the caregiver,* as for instance: reproaching the patient for his clumsiness or disturbing behavior; sending the patient out of a room where he is not supposed to be, which leads to his quickly becoming upset and agitated; giving him assignments which he is no longer capable of carrying out; performing movements with him at too high a tempo and in an aloof manner; suddenly taking hold of him from behind, or pushing him or making him walk backwards.

It is advisable to draw up a 'first aid list' and display it near the telephone, with:
- names, addresses and telephone numbers of doctor and family, the regular caregiver, the ambulance service and hospital;
- office address and telephone number of partner

11. Look for specific disabilities, occurring with specific motions. Some patients may have difficulty with reaching as a result of impaired vision or arm mobility. Others may have difficulty when trying to sit down on account of loss of positional reflexes or inability to recognize a chair. Other patients have difficulty turning around

Preventing falls by special techniques

It is important that the caregiver knows how he can help the patient alter his posture when the patient is himself no longer able to adjust his posture to the demands of the various necessary daily activities.

During the course of the four stages various locomotor problems occur, to which the patient must adjust with the help of his caregiver. The more the locomotor symptoms of the Alzheimer process increase, the more important proper and efficient supporting and lifting techniques become, both for the wellbeing of the patient and for the caregiver's bodily good. Not only does the patient become ever more rigid, he may also resist the caregiver who is trying to help him. Consequently, putting these techniques into practice is not easy. The patient cannot take an active part in letting the movements take place as smoothly as possible. Great demands are made on the physique and the tactfulness of the caregiver. It is important that the caregiver should receive training in physical support and lifting techniques, specifically oriented to the problems of the dementing patient. The following examples serve to illustrate this. It is important for the caregiver to maintain eye contact with the patient and always tell him what is going to happen.

Getting the patient to sit on a chair or on the edge of the bed from the standing posture in stage IIIB.

1. The caregiver approaches the patient from an oblique angle from the front, with his arms outstretched and the palms of his hands uppermost. In response to this inviting gesture the patient puts his hands in those of the helper.
2. The helper grasps the patient's hands and puts them on his own shoulders and supports the patient's elbows in the hollows of his own elbows.
3. Subsequently the helper lays both his hands on the patient's shoulders, so that he has a good grip. The helper and the patient are now standing at an arm's length from one another.
4. The helper makes caressing, steering movements on the patient's shoulders and moves slowly in the direction of the chair, and with his own back towards the chair or bed, using small 'dance' steps and meanwhile humming or singing. Having arrived at the chair or the bed, he slowly turns around with small steps, until the patient is standing with the back of his thighs against the chair or the edge of the bed. Take care! The patient is not able to walk backwards.
5. The helper continues to hold onto the patient by both shoulders and maintains and stimulates contact by making massaging movements with his hands on the patient's shoulders and talking to him in a friendly way. Take care! If you let go of the patient, you have to begin all over again!
6. The helper, with his legs in the stepping position and his knees slightly bent, puts one leg forward, and with his own foot in front of the foot of the patient, and presses his knee, loosely but fixatingly, against the patient's knee.
7. The helper subsequently transfers his own balance to his back leg, so that he is leaning slightly backward, which forces the patient to move his bottom backwards, resulting in his head, knees and hips bending. Take care! The patient is incapable of estimating height, depth or breadth.
8. The helper keeps his own weight on his backmost leg (counterweight) and makes a gently to and fro swaying (tango) movement and slowly gets the patient to sit in this flowing movement.

9. The helper lightly rubs the back of the patient's hand and lower arm, if the latter continues to keep hold of the helper. This loosens the grasp.

It is advisable to practise this method of getting from 'standing to sitting' several times with a healthy partner.

Another possibility of getting the patient to sit on the edge of the bed or lie on the bed in stage III B.

1. The helper approaches the patient from an oblique angle from the front, with his arms outstretched and the palms of his hands uppermost. Through this inviting gesture the patient lays his hands in those of the helper.

2. The helper grasps the patient's hands and puts them on his own shoulders and supports the patient's elbows in the hollows of his own elbows.

3. The helper subsequently puts both his hands on the patient's shoulders, so that he has a good grip. The helper and the patient are now standing at arm's length from one another.

4. The helper makes caressing, steering movements with his hands on the patient's shoulders and moves slowly in the direction of the bed, and with his own back towards the bed, with small 'dance' steps and meanwhile humming or singing. Having arrived at the bed, he slowly turns around with small steps, until the helper and the patient are standing with one shoulder facing sideways to the bed.

5. The helper continues to keep hold of the patient by both shoulders and maintains and stimulates contact by making massaging movements with his hands on the patient's shoulders and talking to him in a friendly way.

    Take care! Letting go of the patient means starting all over again!

6. The helper, with his legs apart and knees slightly bent, now makes slow sideways to and fro movements with the patient and in the meantime brings the patient closer to him (fixation).

7. The helper gradually transfers his bedwards-pointed hand from the patient's shoulder to the latter's bedwards-pointed elbow and grasps the elbow.

8. With his other hand, which is still resting on the patient's shoulder, the helper now exerts slight pressure backwards during the swaying to and fro movements and moves his own feet a quarter turn, so that he is now facing the bed.

9. In a flowing movement the helper tilts the patient first slightly sideways in the direction of the bed and in the tilting action steers the patient's trunk into the sitting position or straight into the lying down position.

10. The patient now pulls his legs into bed himself and lies down and moves into the position of his choice.

11. The helper gently rubs the back of the patient's hand and lower arm, if he continues to hold onto the helper, and talks to him in a friendly manner.

    Take care to avoid both tilting into bed together!